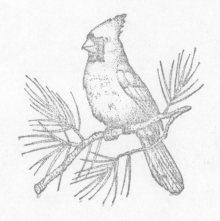

ALSO BY LONNY SHAVELSON

Toxic Nation: The Fight to Save Our Communities from
Chemical Contamination (with Fred Setterberg)
I'm Not Crazy, I Just Lost My Glasses
Personal Ad Portraits

A CHOSEN
DEATH

The Dying Confront Assisted Suicide

by Lonny Shavelson

PHOTOGRAPHS BY LONNY SHAVELSON

UNIVERSITY OF CALIFORNIA PRESS
Berkeley · Los Angeles · London

University of California Press
Berkeley and Los Angeles, California

University of California Press, Ltd.
London, England

First Paperback Printing 1998

Published by arrangement with Simon & Schuster Inc.

Designed by Liney Li

Manufactured in the United States of America

1   3   5   7   9   10   8   6   4   2

Library of Congress Cataloging-in-Publication Data

Shavelson, Lonny.
    A chosen death : the dying confront assisted suicide / by Lonny
Shavelson ; photographs by Lonny Shavelson.
        p.   cm.
    Originally published: New York : Simon & Schuster, c1995.
    Includes bibliographical references (p.   ).
    ISBN 0-520-21292-4 (alk. paper)
    1. Assisted suicide—Case studies.   I. Title.
R726.S526   1998
179.7—dc21   97-36928
                                                                                      CIP

CONTENTS

Preface to
the Paperback Edition

———————

S ince the initial 1995 publication of this book, the question
of the right of a terminally ill patient to have help in
hastening his or her death has wound its way to the
Supreme Court, and a decision from on high was duly delivered. The result, I am pleased to announce for this paperback
edition of *A Chosen Death*, was that both sides won.

Patients have been begging for better deaths and, thanks to
changes in medical practice brought about by the Supreme
Court hearings, they will have them.

On January 6, 1997, the day before the court heard arguments for and against the legalization of physician-assisted suicide, the American Geriatrics Society, a group of 6,000 health
providers who focus on serving the needs of the elderly, joined
forty other associations (including the American Nurses Asso-

ciation and the American Association of Retired Persons) to announce that they will no longer tolerate poor pain control and other indignities of inadequate care for the dying.

Where were these groups before this issue went to the Supreme Court? Did the dying have to threaten to kill themselves before those organizations joined up to fight for better care at the end of life?

The American Medical Association (opposed to physicians ever hastening any patient's death, because "doctors are healers, not killers") argued to the Supreme Court justices that dying patients need improved pain control, not lethal prescriptions. A few months later, the AMA produced a plan to teach better pain relief techniques in medical schools. We can thank the Supreme Court battle for that kindness.

In its lengthy preparation for the court hearings, The Death With Dignity National Center, a coalition of organizations working toward legalization of physician aid-in-dying, opened an intense dialogue with hospice workers. The goal of both groups was to improve end-of-life care, and so reduce the demand for assisted suicide. Hospice workers, in turn, reconsidered their unbelievable claim that they can make all deaths comfortable. They now admit that in some circumstances, when the agony is severe, they resort to sedating patients into a coma— about as close as you can get to assisted suicide without crossing the line.

Groups of physicians and health care administrators, in more than one hundred "friend of the court" briefs representing opinions from that of the American Hospital Association to the American Medical Students Association, were forced to scrutinize the effects of managed care on end-of-life decisions: Is it cheaper to let people die? Even less expensive to assist them in suicide? And does the common and legal practice of disconnecting life-support machinery carry similar risks of abuses to those so fearfully pointed out in legal briefs against the legalization of doctor-assisted suicide?

Physicians across the country have re-examined the fee-for-service system as well: Do doctors make more money by keeping patients alive, long after they cry out for the mercy of death?

Health care providers who argued that the court should not allow physicians to offer dying patients the option of hastening their deaths, were pushed to produce concrete plans of better alternatives for those patients who suffer beyond their limits as life approaches its end. These plans are now translating into real changes in pain control and hospice care for the dying. If the trend continues, assisted suicide (legal or not) will be a less-requested option.

In Washington, a disability rights group called "Not Dead Yet" protested on the steps of the Supreme Court, enlightening us to their reality—that we often confuse disabilities with terminal illnesses. Not Dead Yet members feel threatened by any decision that would legalize assisted suicide, fearing that people with disabilities will be offered quicker deaths instead of better lives. We have heard their message.

With each side of the assisted suicide debate forced to make their most well-reasoned points to the court, we have gained new insights as to how dying patients are both treated and tortured as they near death. And both sides reached an indisputable common ground: Whether assisted suicide is legal or not, better care for the dying is crucially needed.

On June 26, 1997, the nine justices of the Supreme Court ruled unanimously that terminally ill patients have no constitutional right to a physician's aid in hastening their deaths. But they agreed that there was no reason an individual state could not declare such a practice to be legal, effectively tossing the question back to the fifty-two states.

And now that the battle is over in the chambers of the court, we can judge the effect it had on all participants, forcing them to accept fundamentally reasonable principles, and to find common ground:

• Hospice care should be universally supported and available, so that more dying patients can live their final days in home hospices, not intensive care units.

• People with disabilities should have assistance to better lives, not easier deaths.

• All patients in pain at the end of life must have access to adequate amounts of pain medications, including narcotics, to be administered by practitioners trained and experienced in treating the widest range of suffering.

In other words, if we are to move past the present-day raging epidemic of cries for assisted suicide, we must realistically provide comprehensive and thorough care to those who are dying.

We have heard the voices of the dying, the disabled, the uninsured and the poorly treated. We have listened and will respond to their needs.

The justices of the Supreme Court handed back to each individual state the decision whether to legalize assisted suicide for terminally ill patients. But few who watched the arguments closely are now willing to prognosticate as to which side will prevail in this new forum. Based on what I saw at the Supreme Court hearings, I'm glad to do so: The patients will win.

Lonny Shavelson
Berkeley, California
August, 1997

Preface

Two years before I was born, my mother sat at the bedside of her fifty-nine-year-old dying mother. After her second heart attack, my grandmother had become so weak she was unable to leave her bed. That year, 1949, she remained at home under an oxygen tent, too short of breath to lift a spoon to feed herself. For reasons my parents to this day claim they don't understand, my grandmother, the matriarch who helped the entire family escape the pogroms in Russia in 1910, stopped talking. The only words she uttered were in Yiddish, always in the middle of the night. *"Rateve mir, rateve mir"*—"Save me, save me," she'd yell. My grandfather, my father and my mother could not sleep at night during the ten months of my grandmother's nocturnal anguish; in the daytime, they endured her determined silence.

The family physician, a Polish immigrant who had known my grandmother for years, arrived at the house daily for ten months, to treat the heart failure that kept her constantly short of breath. Death was only days away, he kept telling my parents and grandfather. No one spoke to my grandmother about it; the family did not believe the doctor's prediction. "I'm going to make her better," said my mother, explaining her unceasing bedside vigil.

At the end of this exhausting ten months, my grandmother was suddenly blinded by the effects of a stroke. Barely able to breathe, bedridden for nearly a year, willfully not speaking, she was now also unable to see. Still not uttering a word, she swung her arms about, searching for people she heard in the room, then collapsed into a stupor from the strain of the activity, and the terror.

Her doctor arrived. My father greeted him, then said he needed to leave for a moment to go to the store. "Stay," said the doctor.

My mother was in the bedroom with my grandmother. "I was holding Mom's hand," she recalled, "and I could feel the pulse at her wrist going lickety-split." The doctor stood at the bedside with her. He said little, then drew up a syringe and gave my grandmother an injection. He remained in the room. Ten minutes later, my mother stared at him. "Her pulse has stopped," she said. "Yes, I know," the doctor replied. "I carried on like a lunatic," remembered my mother. "Then they took me from the room."

"What happened?" she later asked her brother. "Dr. Berger did the best thing he could for Mom," surmised my uncle, explaining that the injection had probably been the cause of her death, and originating a family story that has since grown to mythical proportions. "All I knew," my mother told me years later, "was that Mom wasn't suffering anymore."

• • •

In the household of my childhood, my mother simply assumed it would be appropriate for me, the son, to help end her life when she decided she was ready. As a child, I thought this was a common family arrangement.

Plans for me to become a doctor had started with the benign message "It's good to help people." Yet childhood discussions of stethoscopes and doctors' plushly carpeted offices segued rapidly into talks of my finding a cure for my mother's suffering from her chronic illness. Bedridden with Crohn's disease, an inflammation of the bowel accompanied by infections, fevers and weakness, my mother was also, I now understand, severely depressed. And for me the childhood struggle between independence and family responsibility became hopelessly tangled in questions and fears about illness and suffering, and the devastating emotional effects they could have on a family. My preordained role in life, it seemed, would be to find a cure for my mother's disease. Failing this, if she became severely ill, my mother asked me to give her a fatal intravenous injection of potassium chloride. I was fourteen years old.

"How could you even dare?" my father said to my mother in a family conversation this year, when I told him for the first time that she had asked me to kill her when I was fourteen. She'd made the same request of him, he confessed, but he misinterpreted it as a discussion about some future eventuality. "Would you put me out of my misery?" she had asked him back then. "There's no reason to talk about it now," replied my dad, ending the discussion.

When my father refused to talk to my mother about her wish to die, she had turned to me. "You were my only source, Lon," she tells me today. "I would have jumped out the window right then if I'd had the courage. But I needed help—and you were the logical one to do it."

My father had missed the fact that it wasn't Mom's illness that brought on her death wish. My mother's thoughts of suicide came from her long-term depression (to which no doubt her illness had contributed), made intolerable when my sister and I were old enough to recognize and resent her continued distress and sorrow.

From the time I was fourteen to today, my mother, now seventy-five, has been in and out of remissions of both her disease and her depression. Having endured the worst of times and recovered, she still holds at bay her final request for me to help in her suicide. But as old age compounds her suffering from illness and depression, the time will undoubtedly come when she decides there is no turning back, no hope for improvement. And she will again recall the source of relief of her own mother's suffering, and ask me to provide that same relief for her.

"I had two children and a husband," she tells me today, remembering her request of her fourteen-year-old son to help in her suicide—the first of oft-repeated but never fulfilled pleas that have now tortured us for twenty-eight years. "I was making everyone miserable," she recalls, "and I wanted to die."

"So you asked me to kill you," I respond now, "and blamed the whole thing on your illness?" But I stop the conversation there—still keeping my secret, that her repeated discussions of suicide, her lack of desire to live coupled with requests for me to kill her, had sucked me into the hole of her depression, leading me at fourteen into two years of grappling with my own plans for suicide.

I left home when I was sixteen. Planning a parent's death, I realized, should be no part of a child's life. In search of relief from my own depression, I put aside Mom's requests for my help in her suicide.

• • •

In 1992, as I was well into a career as a physician and journalist, the question of assisted suicide jumped out at me again. Jack Kevorkian was in the news almost daily. *Final Exit,* a recipe book of overdoses for people with terminal illnesses, hit the *New York Times* bestseller list, and stayed there for eighteen weeks as 520,000 Americans decided they needed to own a how-to manual for suicide. Washington State and the State of California had put initiatives on the ballot to allow physicians to aid in suicides of the terminally ill. Everywhere I turned, it seemed, people were talking about assisted suicide as a possible escape from the extreme suffering that can accompany a prolonged illness.

I had thought my childhood experience confronting euthanasia in the family was aberrant; now, assisted suicide was the topic of kitchen-table discussions in hundreds of thousands of households.

That same year, my father, having survived two heart attacks, went into rapid respiratory failure for unknown reasons. In the hospital's intensive care unit the doctors considered hooking him up to a breathing machine. My dad's X ray showed almost no normal lung tissue. His ability to deliver oxygen to his body was minimal. He hallucinated throughout the night, waking intermittently in a panic, thinking he was dead. I held his hand and stroked his forehead so he'd know he was still alive. When he was awake, he told me about his hallucinations. They were in Yiddish, which he hadn't spoken since childhood. His mind was in Brooklyn, somewhere around 1931 when he was twelve and had helped support his family by shining shoes and selling newspapers. He seemed to enjoy being there, except for the moments of clarity when he assumed these dreams meant he had died.

My father was gasping for air, suffering greatly. At one point, as the doctor threaded a plastic tube into his ailing heart, it stopped pumping—only to recover a minute or so later, for reasons as mysterious as its sudden cessation.

During his rare coherent moments, my father repeated one thing with great clarity: "Don't let me die!" My dad would endure *anything* to live one more day, to tell yet another story to a friend. I sat in awe of my father's tenacity and stamina in the face of this torturous suffocation.

My dad survived what turned out to be a rare reaction to a heart medication he'd been taking. He is alive and well, three years after making the decision to fight on at all costs. Had it been my mother in that hospital bed, she would have begged me for the overdose. But to this day, as her own disease and unhappiness still waxes and wanes, she has managed to put off her final request for death. Yet when the times comes, as it surely will, I know I'll tremendously disappoint her if I don't follow through on my childhood promise to give her the potassium chloride.

In 1992, my boyhood and adolescent struggle with questions of illness and assisted suicide burst into the open and grew raw again. I was stunned by the intensity of debate about Kevorkian, and the enormous public interest in the book *Final Exit*— perhaps the most telling indication of the prevalence of hidden assisted suicides in America. I realized that, secretly, in darkened bedrooms across the country, thousands of parents, children, husbands, wives, sisters, brothers, lovers and friends were deciding whether or not to aid in the death of a loved one. And as the furor of public debate raged on, I faced my own lifelong ambivalence about how to handle the tremendous physical and emotional agony that can be brought on by illness and disease.

By contacting hospices for the dying and other family support organizations, I searched out people who had been forced by impossible circumstances to confront their own personal dilemmas about illness and assisted suicide, people who could not wait for physicians, ethicists, lawyers, and legislators to find answers for them. Through their torment, I began to grapple with my own.

And I might have predicted from the intensity of my childhood experiences that I would leave behind my physician's emotional distance, and my objectivity as a journalist, when I joined this underworld of people making decisions to assist, or not, in the suicide of someone for whom they cared deeply. But I had no idea that I would be led to the deathbed of Renee Sahm—and what I might do when I got there.

LONNY SHAVELSON
January 1995

Chapter One

Plan A:
The Fight to Survive

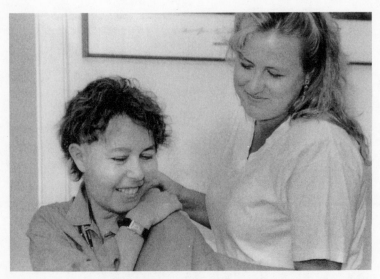

Renee Sahm with her best friend Margie Monson,
soon after Renee's second brain surgery.

T he day Renee Sahm decided to kill herself I was completely unprepared. I shouldn't have been. She had asked me some months earlier to tell her story, and we'd talked about her death on dozens of occasions. I thought I knew what to expect when the moment came. I was wrong.

If there is a gene for survival instinct, Renee Sahm had it. Conceived by middle-aged parents who met in Germany while searching in vain for family survivors of the Holocaust, Renee learned early on about perseverance. As the teenage child of elderly parents, and a Jew in postwar Germany, she developed a self-sufficiency and independence she'd carry through life. At twenty-one, she left for California. "Suddenly everything was up to me," she recalled. "It fit so much better."

Renee found work in the government, researching, designing and lobbying for emergency disaster planning. She dove into the complexity of the job; endless bureaucratic battles merely bolstered her love for a good fight.

Renee's social life was devoted more to activities than people. She sought friendship and adventure by learning to fly small aircraft and in skydiving. She joined a sports-car club and raced around town in a red classic MG. Her love life-followed the same independent course. She was married once, briefly, "mainly for immigration reasons."

Rarely lacking close friends or lovers, Renee still spent most of her time alone in a small suburban home. Her most intense love was reserved for her work as writer and researcher. Her life, she said, was "carefully controlled."

Those life experiences guided Renee's response when, at thirty-six, the first pain hit—a sharp sudden headache that nearly knocked her to the floor. "It was so bad," she remembered, "I dialed 911." Within minutes, the pain was gone. Only then did Renee move from action to emotion. "I was soaked in sweat," she said. "It scared the hell out of me."

Renee "researched the headache." "It was a bureaucratic nightmare," she recalled. "You cannot walk into a hospital, especially a large HMO, and say, 'Excuse me, I had a head-ache.' They told me I was fine." She leapt to the challenge. "After a number of doctors gave the same silly answer," she said, "the fun began, the Renee part." She advised the public relations officer of her HMO that she would see a private neurologist, send the HMO the bill, and tell her friends in the senate all about it. "How about an appointment with our specialist, 8:30 A.M.?" offered the PR man. "How about 8:00?" she responded.

"You know," Renee said, telling me this story five years later, "I was so wrapped up in getting them to pay attention to me, I forgot to worry about what they might say when they discovered what caused the pain."

• • •

A CAT scan showed cancer in her brain. And Renee's response belied the claim that people with terminal illnesses who plan to take their own lives are quitters.

Renee endured painful neurosurgery, radiation, and the nausea, vomiting and hair loss brought on by months of chemotherapy. "God, it all terrified me," she recalled. With these efforts, she halted the cancer for two years. When it grew again, doctors told Renee nothing more could be done. Yet one physician mentioned an experimental program in Sweden that had helped a patient he knew. Unwilling to raise her hopes, he wouldn't say more. So Renee tracked down the patient, con-tacted the Swedish consulate in Chicago, and talked her way into the experimental European program. In Sweden she underwent radical new therapy with a "gamma knife"—a slicing beam of intense radiation. The tumor virtually disap-peared.

Renee's passion for research and planning turned inwards. "This cancer is something that cannot be shared," she said. "With all the friendship, all the support I have, it's in my body only. It's a very solitary experience." The daily work of staying alive—tracking the progress of her cancer with ever more advanced scans and tests, deciding between alternative treatments, studying, meeting with doctors—became an obsession that changed Renee's very being. If there is any tragedy to the story of Renee Sahm, it's that she gave up her life in order to live.

In spite of medical successes, Renee's energy and freedom were gone. Her time, previously filled with furious clashes at work followed by weekend flying and skydiving lessons, became centered around home. "It's a pick-up-the-dry-cleaning kind of thing," she said in frustration. "I want to finish this cancer affair and do something else. But it's always the cancer, then the bureaucracy. Having to ask for things over and over is the hardest thing for me—to go out begging for this new treatment, that new test; it tires me so quickly. But if I hadn't taken care of it I would have died long ago."

Renee's strategizing continued: "Plan A," she said, "is to fight like hell to live. Plan B is my suicide, if Plan A fails and the suffering becomes unbearable."

For Plan B, Renee contacted the Hemlock Society, bought and studied the book *Final Exit*, and became as knowledgeable about how to die as she had been about the new medical treatments that allowed her to live. And she agreed to discuss with me the reasons she planned to kill herself.

• • •

When I met Renee, a barely five-foot-tall woman with a soft voice that nonetheless could argue her way out of a New York cab fare, her cancer was in full remission. She felt fine.

Photographs she had taken of beach scenes and swans decorated her house on a quiet tree-lined street. She was dressed, as always, in solid colors, her only adornment a simple lapel pin.

"Why does someone who feels this good, enjoys her life, and has done so well with treatment," I asked, "invite me over to talk about her suicide?"

"I remember a routine checkup two years ago," she began. "I'd been doing so well. When my doctor arrived, I exclaimed happily about her gorgeous yellow dress. I was that unprepared. Then I saw the pain in her eyes. She opened her arms and she held me. 'There's nothing more we can do,' she said."

In spite of her doctor's statement, Renee searched out and found the gamma knife and gained additional years of life. But the agony of surprise she had felt when the doctor pronounced her death sentence left permanent scars. Living or dying, Renee needed to have control.

"I won't face death so unprepared the next time," she told me. "It's not going to surprise me."

Over the next months, Renee and I had dozens of meetings. She became my mentor at thriving in the face of adversity. We'd linger longer after each interview, our friendship growing. I was at her side when she regained consciousness following her second successful neurosurgery, after the tumor had again returned. And I joined in with her other friends when she threw herself a "neurosurgical recovery and birthday party," fifteen days after the surgeon had sewn her skull back together.

Renee settled into a home routine. "It doesn't sound like much to redo a screen door," she told me, "unless you know old wooden screen doors. It makes me feel good to fix it, to just be me for a while, not Renee with cancer."

Over time, Renee and I talked less about cancer and the daily details of Plan A, her fight to live, or even Plan B for her

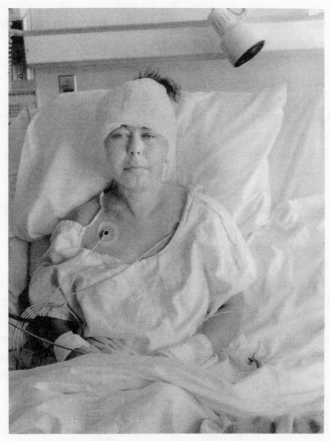

*"Plan A," the fight to survive—
recovering from brain surgery.*

suicide. In spite of her disease, and my own obsessive research into suicide and terminal illness, our friendship grew to include other parts of our lives. By February 1993 she'd been doing so well for such a long time, and we were talking so infrequently about suicide, that we went for a congratulatory lunch and, laughing, abandoned the project and toasted our friendship. Renee Sahm seemed a long way from dying.

• • •

At 11:30 P.M., one month later, I turned on my answering machine: "Lonny, I must talk to you." I had never before heard Renee's voice tremble. "Lonny," she said, "please come."

The tumor had spread outside her brain, to a lymph gland in the neck. "How amazing," she told me, "to finally feel it, to hold the cancer in my hand—to know it's really there."

Five years after receiving her fatal diagnosis, Renee began to die. "Maybe through me, Lonny," she said, "you'll get a good hit of what it's really like."

A week later, Renee was found at home, barely conscious, thrashing about in confusion. She was taken to the hospital's hospice unit. In the adjacent bed was an emaciated elderly woman at the edge of death.

When I visited Renee there, she opened her eyes, saw me, and tried to speak. She could barely whisper. "What a nice face to wake up to," she said. I cried. Her next words were more firm: "Untie me." Renee was strapped to the bed rails. "I woke up in the middle of the night," she explained, "and started yelling to let my dog in. Then I realized where I was and insisted I had the right to go home. That's when they tied me down." I called for the nurse to untie her.

Renee drew my head close to her face. "Get the pillow from my house," she said, "and my mohair blanket." I brought these. She grasped the blanket, put the pillow behind her head, lay back and grinned. "I need some piece of *me* here."

I sat with Renee's best friend, Margie, and tried to piece together what had happened. The tumor in Renee's neck created pressure that made it difficult for her to swallow. At home, she had briefly stopped sipping liquids. Then she became too dehydrated, weak and confused to remember to drink at all. It spiraled downhill from there.

In the hospice, with better liquid intake, Renee regained her strength and clarity of thinking. But it was apparent that she was no longer safe alone at home. Even when her dehydration had been treated, Renee was occasionally confused. Her weakness progressed. And we were sure the tumor had also spread inside her brain.

"I keep losing my thoughts in the middle of a sentence," Renee told Margie and me. "I have to search for what I was talking about. It's like a pearl earring I've misplaced somewhere." She puzzled out the feeling. "It's such a relief when I find the thought again."

A few days later, barely able to walk, and against the advice of friends, nurses, and physicians, Renee left the hospice unit and went home.

"Renee," I said, "your getting sick this quickly sneaked up on us. It's been so long since we've talked about your plan for suicide. I don't know what you're thinking now."

Renee laughed, then stared at the wall. "I guess there are still surprises, Lonny. I have no Plan B."

Thinking she had slipped into confusion, I tried again, as gently as I could. "Renee, we've talked about Plan B for the past year and a half."

"I know. All this talk about *Final Exit,* suicide, medications. But you see, I never really believed I'd die from this." She paused, wanting to be sure I understood. "Plan A is shot to pieces. And I'm too weak to organize Plan B now, do the research, go to different doctors, lie to get enough sleeping pills. I'm stuck." I sensed what was coming next, and I too had

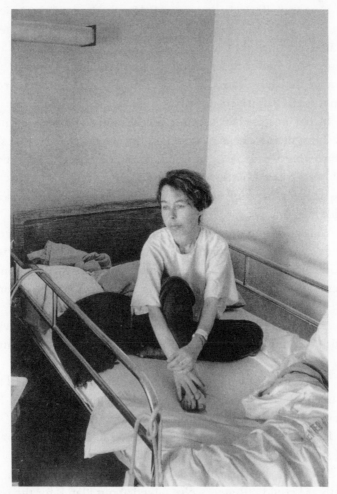

In the hospice unit, soon after Renee
was untied from the bed rails.

not thought through my plans. "Lonny," said Renee, "I'm going to need your help."

· · ·

On a warm spring afternoon a few weeks later, Margie and I sat at Renee's bedside at home. Renee was down to seventy-nine pounds, unable to walk, intermittently confused. She was fading quickly. Yet for unpredictable periods of time, stimulated by visits from friends, Renee would become alert and talkative, clear-minded.

Like me, Margie felt the need to know Renee's thoughts on Plan B. Did she now want to let the matter drop, to sink toward a natural death, however it might occur? "I'm not sure how long you'll be able to communicate with us," Margie said, quite bluntly. "Can you tell us what you want?"

Renee became annoyed. She refused to talk about suicide or her death. "I see my doctors next week," she said. "I want them to go over my entire case. They've told me I was dying before, and we found something to do." Renee had been to death's door and back four times in five years. Why acquiesce now?

Margie and I walked to a nearby park. "Renee has made it clear," said Margie, "she's not ready to die."

"I don't know if she has that choice anymore," I responded. "But her thoughts about suicide aren't there today. After years of coherent philosophy about euthanasia, what counts is what she feels now."

At home, I reviewed my notes from over forty interviews with Renee. Throughout, she was clear that she did not want to prolong an agonizing death. "I'm terrified of the last few weeks with brain cancer," she'd told me. "Pain. Delirium. Hopelessness. Dependence. I abhor dependence."

Yet there were hints of ambivalence all over the place; I had missed every one of them. "I believe that by suicide," Renee had said, "I'm romanticizing my own death, so it will be as big a deal to everyone else as it is to me." Another time: "I'm trying to test my friends, to see who will be there for me." Yet again: "I'm creating a story for myself, to show I'm in control—to ace Suicide 101!"

And most significantly, Renee had told me, warned me: "I have a pit bull personality. I'll come back kicking and screaming when I need to."

There was no Plan B.

• • •

Renee's confusion slipped into hallucinations. On May 26, the former small-aircraft pilot lay in bed screaming, "WE'RE GOING TO CRASH! PULL OUT NOW, DAMN IT!" She grabbed the bars of the headboard, tugged at imaginary flight levers, cried out when they failed her. When she sensed the ground approaching, her shriek was bloodcurdling. Helpless, we stood by for hours, listening to her screams, interspersed sporadically by shouts of "SCORPIONS! KILL THEM!"

Then Celia, a close friend of Renee's who'd been away for two years, walked into the room. Though I don't believe in miracles, I know I saw one. Renee looked at Celia, recognized her immediately, and sat bolt upright. Then she burst into tears. "I love you," said Celia. Renee became coherent. She and Celia giggled, told stories, hugged, stroked each other's hair. In the heat of their friendship, the hallucinations vanished. It was a pajama party, not a deathwatch. Margie, Renee's friend John, and I, having watched days of Renee's agonizing dementia, sat in awe.

Then Renee shocked us all. She introduced me to Celia, saying, "Lonny is writing a book about suicide. I'm in it. It's for you too. Because you have to know why I'm going to do it."

"Renee," I said cautiously, "we didn't know you were still thinking about suicide."

Renee addressed Celia, who disapproved of suicide under

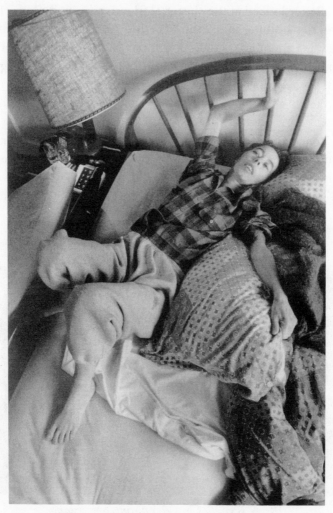

Renee's confusion slipped into hallucinations.

any circumstances. "Three separate terminal diagnoses," she began, "and I continued to live. But this time—no, it's enough. I can't keep running anymore. I can't focus my eyes. I can't drive my car. My God, I can't even walk. I fought this thing hard. I have no options left."

Renee looked at the cluster of friends surrounding her bed. "There's nothing after this. Whether I do the suicide or not, the way I am now is the best I will ever be. But I'm afraid of the finality. My death can't be undone." She looked around again. "I'll do it tomorrow," she said. "Suicide tomorrow."

• • •

As Renee fell asleep, John, Margie, Celia, and I filed silently into the living room. "She didn't mean it," I began. There was a simultaneous sigh of relief.

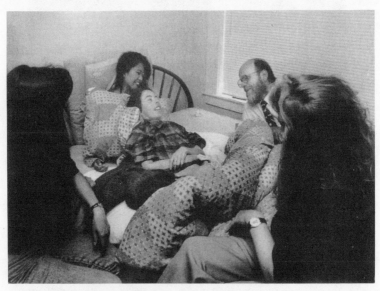

Renee is cradled by Celia during conversation
with friends Lorna, John and Margie.

"I'm not convinced she wants to do it," said Margie. "She's feeling the pressure of what she's told us for the last four years."

John spoke slowly. "There's been no lessening of Renee's

intellectual commitment to suicide. But her spirit's the same old Renee, grasping at every possibility to live. I don't think she realizes she'll go back to the confusion, and she can't decide anything then."

"Renee talks with her intellect," added Celia, "but she always acts from her gut. When she's ready to die, she'll just peacefully go to sleep."

It was my turn to spend the night caring for Renee. Alone with her in the quiet house, I hoped, but doubted, that Celia would be right. Still, I felt a certain pride in the group's carefulness. In spite of Renee's words, I was convinced we had come to the right conclusion.

Renee called to me throughout the night. The scorpions returned. Her swallowing was so impaired that she choked on her saliva, coughing until she was blue. I lay in the bed next to her; she seemed calmer when she wasn't alone. At 5:00 A.M., she hit me. "Lonny, damn you, get up! We need to talk." Renee was coherent again.

"I really am dying," she advised me. "No more gamma knives—no more ideas. Now we get serious. Help me think, to not float away. I need to understand this disease, one more time, to make the right decisions." I remained quiet. "I want you to tell me all of my options," insisted Renee.

I can only hope I was fair in my descriptions; I had seen a number of cancer deaths. "At any moment," I began, "your brain tumor could bleed. You'd have a flashing headache, and you'd die." Renee was tracking all too well. "Would I be certain to die?" she asked. "No. You could remain in a coma," I said. "You could die suddenly in the middle of this conversation, or you could linger for weeks with hallucinations, possibly pain. I can't predict anything. I don't know."

We talked about each possibility. Renee stayed with the conversation for an hour. Only then did she talk about suicide. She asked me how she might do it, still embarrassed by her lack of Plan B. I pointed out that when she left the hospice, her doctor prescribed morphine for pain; twenty-four hundred milligrams of liquid morphine sat in a bottle in her medicine chest.

Renee had me describe her death if she were to drink all of the morphine—essentially a prolonged sleep followed by cessation of breathing. But I couldn't suppress my fears. I knew morphine was fatal in high enough doses. Yet swallowing a lesser amount might only slow Renee's breathing, the lack of oxygen damaging her body and brain without causing her death. The science surrounding suicide for the terminally ill is all anecdotal, and dangerously inexact. Clouded by secrecy, no precise body of medical knowledge has evolved about the best methods for ending the life of someone suffering from a terminal illness. Shockingly little is known about the guaranteed lethal dose of drugs for a person like Renee.

I checked the copy of *Final Exit* on Renee's bookshelf. The lethal dose of morphine for an average-sized man was listed as two hundred milligrams. Renee, seventy-nine pounds and already weakened by her illness, had twelve times the deadly dose on hand. I assured her, and myself, that this must be enough.

But what I didn't speak to Renee about was the most painful paradox to *assisted* suicide: If I would agree to physically administer the lethal dose when she was no longer capable of doing it herself, Renee could live longer. She would not have to guess at this moment whether her anticipated discomfort over the next days or weeks warranted her suicide now. With me as her safety net, to give the lethal dose if she became too weak or hallucinatory to do it herself, Renee could wait to see if she would really need the drug. And she might possibly discover that her natural route to death—now unknown—was acceptable.

With my guarantee to help if her agony became too severe, Renee could live on. Without this promise of aid, if she desired to avoid future *possible* suffering, she must die now, while still mentally and physically capable of taking the overdose.

But while my giving Renee advice on toxic doses is not forbidden, causing her death by my hand, assisting her directly even under these desperate circumstances, is murder. Euthanasia is a capital crime. Any help I provided might cause me to lose my medical license, ruin my career as a journalist, put me in prison. Yet my offer to assist in her death could prolong her life. And it would increase the likelihood that she would not need suicide at all. I suddenly confronted my own indecision about assisting someone to die. And I was not prepared to resolve at that moment what I might do.

I did not mention the option of my assistance to Renee. Nor did I know what I would have said if she had appealed to me then, as her friend, and asked me to help. She didn't.

"Shit," said Renee. "I'm dying. What do I have to wait for?" "Possibly," I said slowly, "some readiness for death—a time when you accept it, rather than saying, 'Shit, I'm dying.' " Renee laughed. "I've read about that, it's not me. I'm dying because I'm forced to die. I hate it." She paused for only a moment. "But I won't risk dying in some of the ways you mentioned. And no more scorpions." She shuddered. "Suicide, tonight."

I believed she meant it. But I'd been through so many circles with Renee I no longer knew what to think. I needed Margie, John, even Celia, to help me und‹ rstand if Renee was sincere. Celia arrived at 7:00 A.M. Margie and John were to visit again that evening. Confused, emotionally and physically exhausted, I left for the day.

When I returned that evening, Celia walked straight by me. "I have to leave," she said. "Renee's going to do it." Renee had spent the day convincing Celia she was ready to die. "I don't agree," Celia told me, "but I'll respect her wishes." John arrived. We discussed the effect of group pressure the night before and decided to talk to Renee individually. "She means it," said John when he left Renee's side. Margie agreed. I walked into Renee's bedroom. "Don't ask me the same questions," she said. "Let's do this."

The intensity of making the decision to die, and the discussions with her friends, had kept Renee clearheaded throughout. My frustration at this trap had no bounds—we supported Renee's decision for suicide because she was still comfortable, clearheaded, and able to do it. In her more confused state the night before, we had not believed the sincerity of her choice. By present-day conventions, Renee had to kill herself while she was still well, or take her chances with whatever a natural death would bring.

Margie was too upset to stay. John offered, but I asked him to go home. "I don't know how this will go," I said. "If there are any questions about Renee's death, John, all you'll be able to say is 'I don't know.'" Renee specifically asked me to stay—she did not want to die alone.

"No more good-byes," Renee insisted after John left. "I've done that with the others." I remained silent. I wanted to do nothing to interfere with this final time she had to herself, the last moment to change her mind.

It took only minutes for her to sip the liquid morphine. She also drank a number of shots of vodka—the effect of alcohol greatly enhances morphine's lethality.

It was 8:00 P.M. Renee was asleep within minutes. Her head fell sideways, hair scattered over the pillow, eyes closed. She never moved from this position. Soon her breathing slowed. A flicker of movement remained above her collarbone, an artery pulsating below her nearly transparent skin. The lethal dose wouldn't reach her brain for hours. I sat, watching Renee, feeling the pain of remembering too much.

By midnight, my breathing matched Renee's—a slow, steady rhythm. Waiting. My torture was tremendous.

At 6:00 A.M., the dawn light illuminated the room. I had not slept. Renee still breathed, shallowly. Her pulse was not diminished.

I was horrified. With the arrival of the sun, our closed world was broken. Renee appeared to be surviving the overdose. It was the worst of our fears. We had talked about failed suicide so many times over the past year, but I had not brought it up again before she took the morphine. I'd been so sure it would be enough. I began to cry.

Had the decision for suicide been a grave mistake, driven by years of intellectual commitment that, in the end, was completely overwhelmed by Renee's will to live on? Was this, her continued breathing, Renee's final magnificent display of her fight to survive? Deeply comatose from the overdose, could she somehow have changed her mind? "I want to live," she had told me. But that choice had been stolen from Renee long before she swallowed the morphine.

The sun shone brightly on Renee's bed. Her breathing was barely apparent, her lips had been blue for too many hours. If I had been sure she'd remain in a peaceful coma, for however long, I might have rested more easily. But I had seen the common consequences of brain damage from oxygen deprivation—a demented thrashing about that can last indefinitely. I agonized over my failure to offer to assist Renee in her suicide. I could have provided for her the guarantee of a comfortable death, and so the paradox of a longer life. Had I done that, Renee would be free from this disastrous ending in which she was now trapped.

Final Exit, opened to the section on morphine, lay by Renee's bed. The author, Derek Humphry, advises a fail-safe backup, in case an overdose causes unconsciousness without death. "I want to emphasize the necessity of the plastic bag in self-deliverance," wrote Humphry. Barbaric, I had thought, and still do.

"Is this what you'd want?" I babbled at Renee's side,

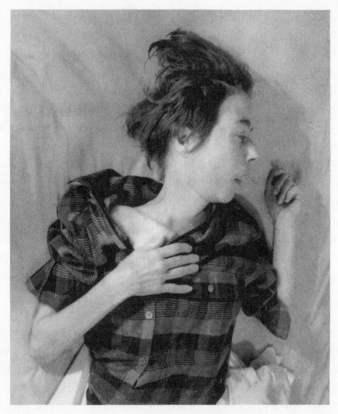

At 6:00 A.M., the dawn light illuminated the room.
Renee still breathed shallowly.

thinking of Humphry's calmly put recommendation. I had no way to know what Renee would want. For all our talks, our friendship, for all our sincerity, we had not made adequate plans. I had no medical tools with me. And even if I did have the right equipment, an overdose by injection would be detectable by the authorities, putting me in great jeopardy.

The hospice nurses, I thought, would be here soon. Renee would be taken to the hospital to linger on, suspended in this state, or worse.

I remembered a story about Renee skydiving from a friend's airplane. "She was so small," said Celia, "that when the parachute approached the ground there wasn't enough weight to pull it down that last few feet. So there was Renee, dangling in the air, her feet running as if she were about to touch the ground, but never making contact. And she just floated across the field like that, feet spinning, laughing away."

I found a plastic bag and sat on Renee's bed, mumbling about her choices, her risks. And I thought of mine. And about the trust she'd had in me.

For families, lovers and friends of people who died in anguish, those who have faced, as I did, the agony of deciding whether or not to help a loved one suffer less—to actually suffocate them—the most difficult part is the loneliness.

We live in torment if we acted; we agonize if we did not.

Either decision would have been—and has become—my life's worst nightmare. Under today's laws, if I were to write that the following scenario actually did happen, I would be confessing to murder and could spend my life in prison.

• • •

I smoothed the hair back from Renee's brow. Cradling her head in my hands, I brushed against the hard tumor just under the soft skin of her neck. *How amazing to finally feel it, to know it's really there,* she had said.

I slipped the black plastic bag over Renee's head, and tucked it into her shirt at the neck. For two minutes, the bag rose and fell with her breathing. Then all was still.

• • •

Sitting by Renee's unconscious body, plastic bag in hand, I had ceased being a writer, or a physician. Nor was I still the child of a depressed and invalid mother who had gained peace from my potential role as her savior. I was a man who had befriended a woman who was dying, as she had befriended me. From some mysterious merger, sitting by Renee's comatose body, I had reached my decision.

But I was not alone that morning with Renee Sahm. I was with hundreds of other families who have faced the anguish of similar dilemmas, in hiding, inexperienced and without adequate guidance. Individually, and now in conversations with each other, we have puzzled through our personal decisions about assisting, or deciding not to, in hastening the death of someone who is desperately ill. But in the harsh, secretive reality of each death, we have been forced to decide, and to act, alone.

And in our conversations we have arrived at one common thought. That this is not how it should be.

Chapter Two

The Moving Line
in the Sand

R enee Sahm had been only seven months from her death when she turned on the TV one evening in late October 1992, at the height of her effort campaigning for the passage of the California ballot initiative, Proposition 161, that would legalize physician assistance in the suicides of people who were terminally ill. At the end of the first commercial, Renee slammed the TV off and was soon banging around the kitchen in a rage.

"Jim Curly was diagnosed with terminal cancer," the announcer's somber voice intoned. Then Jim himself was on the screen. "I thought I was going to die. And until you get in that position, there's no way that it's describable." Jim paused long enough for a banner headline to flash on the TV: PROPOSITION 161 WOULD HAVE KILLED JIM CURLY.

"I didn't want to die," continued Jim, "and I'm glad that proposition wasn't around for me. 'Cause you get so depressed that I might have been stupid enough to say, alright, give me that needle. And I wouldn't be here talking to you people today." Jim's face froze in a still frame on the television. His voice continued. "I would want you and I would want everybody to vote no on 161."

Renee slammed a coffee filter into its holder and waited impatiently for the cup to fill. "God, I hate that, that . . ."—she spilled the coffee, angrily searching for the right words—"willful ignorance. They won't say what it's really like. They presume your doctor tells you at two o'clock you have cancer, and at two-thirty you say, give me a shot to put me out of my misery."

She sat down, placing the coffee cup on her living room table beside her, her voice now calmed to its usual softness. Renee sipped from the cup, then looked up. "That's just not it," she said quietly.

For Renee, who had fought as hard as she could to stay alive while campaigning with equal fervor to make it legal for her doctor to help her die, Jim Curly's commercial was completely off base. But though Renee insisted on her personal freedom to choose the way she might die, there must be Jim Curlys out there who might give up too easily, if tempted. Renee had held suicide as the last resort, her final option in defeat. Yet someone else might just throw in the towel and tragically opt for suicide before the fight had even begun.

Renee had argued for the right to assistance in her suicide. Did others have an equal right not to be tempted by the ease with which they could have this same aid? Would the availability of legalized assisted suicide, as the banner headline in the commercial had claimed, really have been responsible for the death of Jim Curly in a fit of depression?

Pierre Nadeau, a circus trapeze artist dying of AIDS, would unknowingly reveal an answer to this question.

• • •

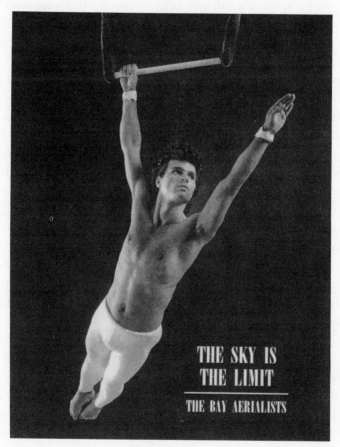

THE SKY IS
THE LIMIT
THE BAY AERIALISTS

Pierre Nadeau

Pierre and Lynn Nadeau stood amid the crowd in the long chandeliered hallway of Davies Hall, the performance of the San Francisco Symphony at an end. The couple hesitated before moving into the rainy evening.

Lynn spotted a cab and made a run for it. Pierre stood by the taxi as she wished him good night. She was heading home to their child; the night was still young for Pierre. But the man with the boyishly handsome magazine-model looks was getting soaked. Lynn offered her umbrella through the car's open window. Pierre inspected it closely, affectionately touched Lynn's face, handed back the umbrella, and without a word walked off into the rain.

"The umbrella, of course, was brown," Lynn told me later, trying to explain why Pierre was ready to commit suicide so soon after the first blemishes of AIDS had become visible on his skin. "A soaking cold rain was OK for Pierre," she said. "An umbrella that clashed with his outfit was simply"—she paused, searching for the words he might use—". . . not acceptable."

People die the way they live. I heard this many times from those who struggled for a simple answer to my prying questions about their planned suicides. "If you understood my life," they'd say, "you'd understand my death."

On February 27, 1992, I phoned Pierre Nadeau in room 617 at Kaiser hospital in San Francisco. Word had reached me that he was intent on killing himself—and soon. But on this first contact with Pierre he was so uninterested in conversation that I'd been taken aback by his request for me to come interview him. Had I known about his life, this invitation as he neared death would not have caught me off guard.

Pierre Nadeau, thirty-two-year-old trapeze artist extraordinaire, lived for the attention of others.

"It's sadder to see Pierre now, more than anyone I know," his friend Darrel had told me. "He was an aerialist in the circus—with a beautifully perfect performer's body that made you gasp when he swung through the air with sleek, smooth movements."

That February in 1992, when I visited Pierre in the hospital, it was clear he was ready to die. It was equally apparent that he was not yet very ill.

Pierre was a grouch. He had always been a grouch, I learned from his friends and family. And from the way it seemed that day, he would die the same way. But Pierre was an intensely well loved grouch. And no matter what he told me about his soon-to-be suicide, this fact would delay his death.

"What do you do with your days, Pierre?" asked Clarissa Ramstead, the hospice nurse with special training in the care of people who are dying. Pierre did not respond. "Do you read?" No answer. "Do you like television?" Silence. Clarissa opened the door to leave the room. "I stare at the walls," Pierre said to her back as she made her exit.

"Oh God," thought Clarissa. "One more person who doesn't even want to talk with me. I just don't want to deal with this." "Very depressed, angry," wrote Clarissa in Pierre's nursing chart. "Wants to be left alone."

But Clarissa went back, time after time. "He'd be lying in bed with the curtains closed, and he'd answer all my questions with just one word," she said. "God, I knew he was upset about the disease, the loss of his body image. You know what a beautiful man he was, what a beautiful body he'd had. When Pierre lost this, it seemed there was nothing left. But as his hospice workers, we somehow had to break through this depression. He had so much else to live for."

"The KS is growing," Pierre told me, showing the AIDS-related purple cancer blotches on his skin, the Kaposi's sarcoma. "Since October, it's one thing after another," he said in disgust.

Pierre pointed to the book *Final Exit* displayed clearly on his bedstand. "I can't move, I can't do anything," he exclaimed as he climbed without difficulty into the high hospital bed. "In June of last year," he said, "I flew the trapeze in Paris. Today, I am here. There is nothing left of me." Pierre sighed. "So I'm going to kill myself."

• • •

"Many so-called right-to-die cases are complicated by depression, anger, and hostility," wrote George Howe Colt in his thorough exploration, *The Enigma of Suicide.*

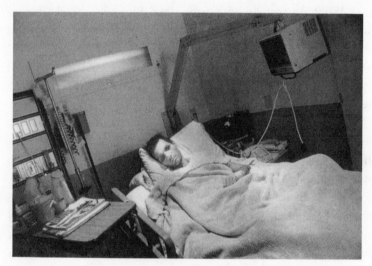

Pierre at Kaiser hospital, February 1992.

The possibility that psychological depression lay at the root of their thoughts of suicide came up for each terminally ill person with whom I spoke. Virtually everyone with a terminal illness who decides to take their life (and many who decide not to) fits the clinical guidelines that would allow a psychiatrist to label them depressed.

Yet the depression of someone with a terminal illness is complexly different from the classical psychological illness.

"I take the word 'depression' very seriously," Renee Sahm had told me during a period of months where she barely left her house, although she felt physically well. "I used to take so much joy in nurturing a plant that needed extra attention," she recalled. "This week, I didn't even water the garden. But damn it, I have a right to be depressed. I'm upset about the cancer. And I'd much rather work through that, meet it head-on, than sign a release form and take Prozac, or whatever the latest pill is."

Two months later, Renee's mood remained dim. "Depression is such a serious condition," she decided. "This lethargic feeling affects every aspect of my life. And I've let it get the upper hand." Renee finally did try Prozac. And she saw a therapist. "How do I put the last four years together into one neat package and get on with my life?" she asked as she made a slow recovery. "The cancer *must* have done tremendous emotional damage. Nobody can be that tough."

Yet at no time during the months of Renee's darkest clinical depression did she talk about using suicide to end it. Plan B, suicide, was reserved for relief from the physical illness that would one day consume her life. Renee didn't even consider suicide as a response to her depression.

For Pierre, the opposite appeared true. Depression seemed the chief motivator in his desire to die. He was not in significant pain. And though he could no longer fly the trapeze, he had the physical strength to walk around, leave the house, visit friends. He had gone to the hospital with a fever from an infected kidney—cured by a thin plastic tube inserted in his back to drain the infection. Unfortunately, the tube had to remain in place to prevent future infections. Yet Pierre was not debilitated by plastic tubes; it was pure unhappiness that had knocked him down. And he was ready to kill himself because of it.

The idea of legalizing euthanasia and assisted suicide does not extend, for the majority of advocates, to helping people kill themselves to avoid unhappiness. Laws allowing physician assistance in suicide will have to deal with situations like the one in which Pierre was foundering, where depression was more the reason for his desire to die than his present physical illness. But people with terminal illnesses who are depressed and desire to die are reacting to different circumstances and should be evaluated in a different light from those who are physically healthy yet still suicidal.

"One of the main justifications for suicide prevention among the young," wrote suicide expert George Howe Colt, "is that their problems are usually temporary and their judgment of them often skewed by depression. For the older person considering suicide, however, depression may be temporary, but loss of movement, vision, hearing, of friends and career, is often irreversible."

"I feel like I'm ninety years old," said Pierre. "And it's not going to get any better."

But would Pierre's suicide at this time be justified by his *future* severe infirmity from AIDS, by the inevitable progression of his ailments? Was his mental anguish this early in the face of a terminal illness reason enough for Pierre to kill himself?

The key, for Pierre and others who are ill, is in whether or not all options for improvement have been exhausted. If someone in physical pain from a terminal illness has not yet been offered pain-relieving medications, their suicide would be premature. The same seemed true in the case of Pierre's depression. There had not been enough of an attempt to break through it, by visits from friends, time with family, physical activity, therapy, possibly antidepressant medications.

Yet some experts examining the issue of physician assistance in suicide have come to extreme conclusions about the role played by depression. "When a terminally ill patient contemplates suicide," writes Dr. Nicholas Pace, who teaches medicine at New York University, "it usually means he or she is suffering from an irrational thought process, characteristic of a major clinical depression." This claim fails to separate the depression that accompanies illness from other types of depression that might lead to "irrational" thoughts of suicide. Renee Sahm, depressed about her illness and the way it had changed her life, also had rational and clearly thought out ideas about how she wanted to die, including assistance in suicide.

Dr. Timothy Quill, a physician who for eight years directed a hospice for the dying, and wrote the book *Death and Dignity*, has come to a different conclusion from Dr. Pace. "To think that the yearning for death by some incurably ill, suffering patients can always be relieved by proper recognition and treatment of depression is a gross oversimplification," writes Dr. Quill.

Both Dr. Quill and Dr. Pace are correct in their understanding of the role of depression in someone's request for a prompt, assisted death; but their conclusions are valid for different patients at different times. There is simply no place for generalizations about people who choose suicide when confronted by the suffering of a fatal illness. Patients must be understood individually, in all of their complexity, to comprehend whether they are depressed, sick and suffering, or most likely some intricate combination that cannot be neatly categorized.

Yet this may be the strongest argument against physician assistance in suicide: Will doctors really spend the time and expend the effort needed to know whether they are dealing with a temporary depression, or a legitimate request to end unbearable suffering? It is alarming to think of a doctor taking a shortcut and helping to kill someone who is briefly upset about his diagnosis, a patient who needs firm reassurance and guidance instead of a lethal injection; and equally appalling if the physician denies a suffering patient's reasoned plea for a comfortable death because the doctor thinks *any* request for suicide, in itself, indicates an irrational thought process.

In the end, it was Pierre's decision whether to kill himself, or to wait to see if his depression would lift; and it is society's decision, in considering new laws for assisted suicide for the terminally ill, whether to help someone in Pierre's situation to end his life.

To me, though, that February when I first met Pierre, the answer seemed intuitively certain: It was too soon for Pierre to die.

• • •

Pierre Nadeau's memories of childhood were filled with images of a magic castle in Quebec. No metaphoric castle, the Nadeau family home was a minareted abode, painted in cartoon colors. To his parents, it was the nightclub from which they earned their living. For Pierre, it was the spired fortress where he, the only boy, and his sisters held forth, where the Québecois came to dance.

When twenty-one-year-old Pierre arrived in San Francisco, the enchantment continued. A gay man of agile grace and beauty, his expectations of adoration were thoroughly fulfilled. San Francisco was a city-castle, steepled in fantasies, embellished by a man who taught him to fly. "The Sky Is the Limit," proclaimed the handbill for Pierre's trapeze performances.

It was a grand fairy tale, broken only by time and place: the '80s, San Francisco. "I was not shocked to discover I was HIV positive," said Pierre.

Pierre had already met and formed a close but platonic bond with Lynn. They decided to live together and have a family, breaking their nonsexual relationship only to conceive a child, Alexa.

Pierre loved Alexa as nothing in his life. Together, they were two kittens at play. Yet Pierre's role as father was performed with less than theatrical zeal. Lynn would care for Alexa while Pierre went off, for weeks at a time, to fly the trapeze.

When he returned home to his daughter, it was to a hero's welcome.

When Alexa was four, she and Lynn moved to Port Townsend, Washington. Pierre remained in San Francisco but visited frequently. He set up a minitrapeze and he and Alexa spent hours together, flying.

The day in February when Pierre decided to kill himself rather than suffer complications of AIDS was five weeks before Alexa's seventh birthday. Alexa knew Pierre was dying. Her schoolteachers, her mother, her friends, and a therapist had all worked to prepare her for his death from AIDS. But no one knew how to prepare Alexa for her father's suicide.

To Alexa, everyone feared, Pierre's suicide before he became seriously ill would seem an act of desertion. Only Pierre could possibly lift from her this added burden.

"I can respect Pierre's desire to die now," said Lynn. "But he has responsibilities for Alexa's feelings as well. And he's not taking care of those."

Pierre reluctantly agreed not to kill himself during the February hospitalization for the kidney infection. He would stay alive until Alexa's visit to San Francisco for her birthday. "But right after that," he said, "I'm going to do it." Pierre paused. "I guess I'll have to talk to Alexa about it first."

On my first visit to the hospital to meet Pierre, his depression was so profound he would barely speak a word. "I'll come back another day," I said, and rose to leave.

"What about the pictures?" Pierre asked softly when I picked up my camera bag. His hand moved from under the covers, finger pointing toward a switch on the wall. His eyes did not move. I flipped the switch. A spotlight used to illuminate patients for medical procedures beamed on over his head. "That's better," said Pierre, bathed in the bright theatrical light. As I began to photograph, Pierre made his first eye contact—with the camera. A moment later, he turned away.

"I'll see you in a few days," he told me. "I want you to document my death."

That day's performance was over. I had no idea what future acts Pierre held in store for me.

• • •

Pierre Nadeau, a gay man with AIDS in San Francisco in 1992, knew that assistance in his suicide would be easily available. Isolated by a society that had rejected them, gays were making their own rules—especially about death and dying. In gay neighborhoods around the country, euthanasia and assisted suicide for people with AIDS became an acceptable norm and an act that was not legally prosecuted. In Los Angeles, AIDS activist Marty James founded an organization called Safe Passages. Before his own suicide on Christmas Day of 1991, James openly assisted in the suicides of fourteen people with AIDS. Yet while Kevorkian was being prosecuted in Michigan for helping in the suicides of heterosexuals, California had turned a blind eye to James' actions.

During those same years, gay men in New York City were thirty-six times more likely to kill themselves than other men between twenty and fifty-nine years old (a low estimate, considering that many AIDS-related assisted suicides went unreported). According to the late reporter Randy Shilts, author of *And the Band Played On,* "Gay men facing AIDS exchange formulas for suicide as casually as housewives swap recipes for chocolate-chip cookies." In a macabre sense, the gay community was writing the rules and performing an experiment with "legitimized" assisted suicide that would show the rest of the country if it could work, or if it would be abused.

"Is that what you'll use to kill me?" Pierre asked Stephen, who had come to visit after he left the hospital. They'd been talking about a friend's recent natural death from AIDS, leaving unused a bottle of morphine prescribed in case he had pain. Stephen had the bottle, along with a slew of potentially deadly pills. It had become a tradition in the AIDS community to bequeath lethal doses of medications to friends who might need them.

"I am *not* going to kill you," Stephen said, his tone hanging carefully between jest and frustration. He glanced at Gordon, the friend who had taken Pierre in to live with him for the duration of his illness.

"Pierre," said Gordon, "you are so lazy you won't even plan your own suicide."

"I have prepared," Pierre replied seriously. "I've given you my power of attorney. I've written my will. And I've told you I want to die."

"And the suicide letter?" asked Gordon.

"We don't have that," Pierre responded slowly, "do we?"

"No," said Gordon. *"You* have to write that."

"Right," said Pierre.

Gordon and Pierre had recited this dialogue so often it came out as a well-rehearsed skit—a twisted Ozzie and Harriet domestic scene. The ease of their conversation had grown from an enduring friendship. Gordon had become Pierre's nurse, cook, mother, father, and unappreciated companion. No one knew what was in it for Gordon to be putting up with Pierre's twenty-four-hour-a-day sullen griping, except possibly saint-hood.

Pierre, dressed in a silk lounging gown, leaned on his gold-tipped cane and twisted toward Gordon. "You aren't going to kill me?" he intoned.

"Let's get this straight, Pierre," interrupted Stephen. "I agreed to help if you were suffering, had decided on suicide, had made definite plans, squared things away with the people you love—and were so sick you couldn't kill yourself without assistance. But I am *not* going to just kill you when you tell me to."

"Read the damn book," added Gordon, pointing to *Final Exit*, not yet opened by Pierre. "Have *some* idea of what this is about. And for God's sake—talk to your daughter."

Pierre nodded absently and wandered to his bedroom. No matter what they told him, he remained certain they'd come through when he needed them.

For the moment, though, he put this aside. Alexa was to arrive for her birthday.

Gordon hung a mobile of crudely crafted paper birds above Pierre's bed. It had come in a package from Lynn that morning. A card said, "Alexa folded love and peace birds into a mobile to brighten your ceiling."

"We have enough stuff in this house," said Pierre. "Take it away."

"We'll hang it for now," replied Gordon. "After she leaves, do what you want with it."

Pierre lay quietly for a moment. "I certainly hope my mood changes before Alexa gets here," he mumbled.

Gordon sat on the edge of the bed. "Lynn is worried," he said, "that if you kill yourself, Alexa will think she wasn't important enough for you to stay alive."

"I'm sure Lynn has told Alexa she is not responsible for my death," responded Pierre.

"You are the magic in Alexa's life," said Gordon. "Only you can tell her why the magic is going to stop."

Pierre closed his eyes, seeming to drift off. Gordon picked up the food tray from the bed and walked from the room.

"Gordon," Pierre called out when his friend reached the door. "It's not my *choice* to die; it's being forced on me. I'd do anything to stay here with her. When Alexa goes back home, what will keep me alive?"

"I'm sure we'll think of something," said Gordon.

• • •

The day before Alexa arrived, Gordon and I met for lunch at the Cafe Flore, an outdoor cafe in the heart of San Francisco's predominantly gay Castro district. It had been Pierre's favorite lunchtime hangout, a place where he would sit alone for only a moment before running into a friend, fan, or potential pickup.

When the purple lesions of AIDS had become visible on Pierre's skin, he'd stopped going to the Flore. He hated the way he looked. And at the Flore, any other man who was HIV positive but had not yet developed AIDS might see in Pierre an image of his own future.

Gordon and I sat in the sun, surrounded by the muscled men of the Castro in tight white shorts and tighter sleeveless T-shirts. The neighborhood around us contained the highest concentration of HIV virus in the country. Yet glancing at the crowd in the hot sun of the outdoor plaza at the Flore, it seemed more a health spa than the nucleus of a lethal epidemic.

Gordon began the conversation with what I thought was a complaint. "Pierre's getting really bitchy about things," he said. "Last night he snapped at Stephen so much, Steve just flipped the finger at him. I said, 'Welcome back, Pierre, it's your old personality again.'"

Gordon explained: "For a while he's been too depressed to even complain. All of a sudden he has this new energy. He's talking about making a cassette tape about himself and Alexa, for her to take home when she leaves." Gordon laughed. "I doubt he'll do it," he said, "but something has changed."

Most notable about my first visit with Pierre and Alexa was how normal everything seemed. Father and daughter were eating breakfast on the sunny balcony of Gordon's apartment, overlooking the San Francisco skyline and out over the blue waters of the East Bay. Lynn was writing letters at the kitchen table. Gordon was cleaning, trying to keep the level of visitor-havoc in his house to a minimum. Nothing seemed unusual— not even the cyclone of energy that burst forth from Alexa.

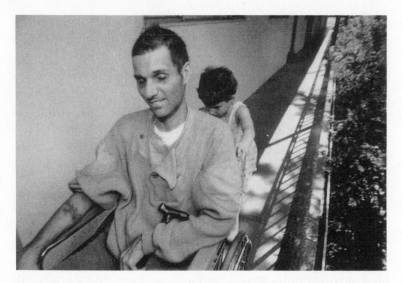

Pierre and Alexa

Alexa was never offstage. Pierre's love, ability, and need to perform had been absorbed by his daughter. And Lynn's dour verbal seriousness, a counterpoint to Pierre's constant physical shenanigans, restrained only a small part of Alexa's unbridled energy.

Lynn introduced me to her daughter as "the man who came to talk to you about your father's death." This was not the way I would have handled the introduction. But Alexa grabbed my hand, pulled me into the room, and climbed on my shoulders to demonstrate back flips onto the couch. Within moments I was just one more of Pierre's friends, a fresh member of the audience.

I liked Pierre much more with Alexa around. His somber pose turned to funny; depressed to playful. Alexa and Pierre romped, joked, attempted dual acrobatics beyond his present physical prowess but well within hers. Yet Alexa learned that day to be gentle with Pierre. He was thinner and weaker than she

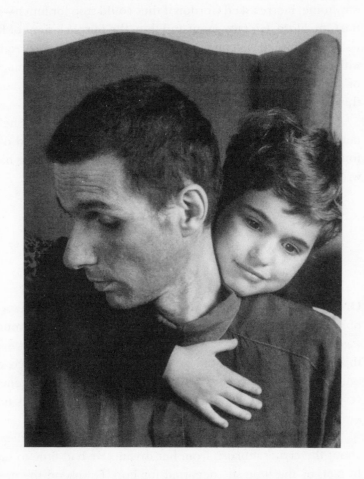

had ever seen him. And he hurt when he was pushed or pulled too hard. Though he was far from death's door, on this visit Alexa discovered that her dad was certainly ill.

Pierre and Alexa went on a clothes-shopping spree. On the way home, Pierre asked Gordon if they could stop for lunch—at the Cafe Flore. His face gaunt and thin, the purple lesions of KS visible in spite of his quick makeup attempt, Pierre was ready, with Alexa's help, to take on the scene at the Flore. The magic of Pierre's earlier life had been transferred to Alexa and, through her, back to him. Almost.

The next day I asked Alexa to show me some drawings she'd made at school during "writing time." She carefully laid out four pieces of colored construction paper upon which she had written and drawn in crayon. They were letters to Pierre.

Dere Daddy I Love You!
iF You WaNt to LiVe You PoabLy weLe Live
iF You DoN't waNt to Live You WON'T.
love Alexa to daddy.

One crayoned drawing showed a tall house with odd-shaped objects hovering over it in the sky. In front of the house was a unicorn, Alexa's favorite animal. From the unicorn's eye, three dark tears fell to the ground. Alexa often dreamed of unicorns. On the day she drew this picture, she had awakened very upset. The unicorn had been crying. Alexa would not say why.

When Pierre came into the room, Alexa told him in detail about the crying unicorn from her dream. He had little to say. In fact, by the time she departed for Port Townsend the next day, Pierre had somehow neglected to talk to Alexa at all about his death, or his pending suicide.

I asked Pierre how this planned conversation with Alexa had worked out. "I'll make her a cassette," he replied.

• • •

With Alexa gone, we waited for Pierre's emotional crash. It never came.

I had wondered if Alexa alone could have been responsible for the entirety of Pierre's spiritual improvement. Pierre didn't just *act* better while Alexa was there—he indeed seemed to be enjoying life again.

"What do you think brought about Pierre's better mood?" I asked Lynn, expecting the "Alexa" answer I'd received from his other friends.

"I haven't a clue," she said. "I've never been dying, so I can only guess. But I imagine that once you actually get right up to the edge and peer over into the abyss, you may want to step back and say, Ooooh!—maybe I don't want to go that way, not right now. Somewhere, something like that has kicked in for Pierre."

Yet Gordon was becoming anxious about the reality of Pierre's improvement in mood. Gordon's own birthday party was planned for the week after Alexa's departure. Late one night, Gordon asked Pierre directly if he would stay alive until his party. "Don't try to get rid of me so fast," replied Pierre. "I'll probably be here for your Christmas party."

In the month after Alexa's departure, Pierre did not once mention the word "suicide."

During that same month, Pierre's physical health declined rapidly. He became gaunt from weight loss. Swollen lymph glands in his groin had grown so large they obstructed the flow of fluid from his legs. His feet and ankles swelled to nearly twice their normal size. It was painful to walk. He also developed a respiratory infection and became short of breath when he tried to move about. Yet while his body had deteriorated, his spirits—and his plans for the future—continued to climb. On May 9, I brought over lunch for Gordon and Pierre and we talked while Pierre sat up in bed.

"I don't know where the depression came from," said Pierre, "because it's not there anymore. It was—an obsession. Day after day I was in the dark. Nothing was worth my being there."

"Why do you think the depression is gone now, and you no longer even mention suicide?" I asked.

"I was very sick then," said Pierre. "Now I'm not. So I feel better emotionally. Who knows? *If* I get sick again, I might get depressed again."

Gordon and I were stunned. Pierre had never been more ill than at that very moment. He was bedridden, short of breath, weak, and wasted. Yet he saw himself to be in better health than when he and I had first met in February.

I pressed on. "Pierre, there's something important for me to know if I'm going to make sense of this whole question of assisted suicide and euthanasia. If in February, when you wanted to kill yourself, the means had been made available, if it had been legal and easier to do—would you have done it then?"

Pierre hesitated, trying to return to his feelings of that time. "No," he pronounced. "Actually, if it was that easy I would wait, because I'd know that I could do it whenever I wanted to. I would have been more tempted to wait. But since it was hard to do—if the chance had come along, I might have taken it." He paused, glancing around his bedroom, then at Gordon and me. "The chance didn't come along. And now I'm here," he said with his sincere half smile, holding back from his performance grin.

Then Pierre became silent, eyes closed. We were unsure if he had dozed off. "What would bring me back to the depression?" he asked suddenly. "Being alive is beautiful. I'm curious to be here one more day. But if I was no longer some part of the world, of society, I don't know if I could stand that. So if I'm at the point where I can't take care of myself, and Gordon has to clean me up every time I shit in my bed . . . I think then I would like to set it up, to have this person and that person here—and at two o'clock, I say good-bye. I would like it to happen that way."

• • •

Stephen Jamison, who holds a doctorate in the sociology of death and dying and specializes in counseling those with terminal illness who are thinking about suicide, calls it the "moving line in the sand." A terminally ill patient draws a line which he simply will not cross. He then arrives at the line, crosses—and draws a new line that he is equally certain he will never cross.

Pierre's line in the sand moved across entire deserts:

Pierre to Lynn, 1990, after visiting a friend sick from AIDS, before he himself had any symptoms: "If I ever get AIDS, I'd just take an overdose and end it all."

February 28, 1992: "I know that someday I'll be plugged in to oxygen all the time. I want to be gone before that."

April 1, 1992, when he was offered chemotherapy to reduce the swelling of lymph glands in his groin: "I'd sooner die than have my hair fall out." (He began the chemotherapy on April 7.)

On multiple occasions from April on: "Diapers. I will not wear diapers and have people clean me up. I'd rather be dead."

On June 29, 1992, Lynn and Alexa came to care for Pierre while Gordon was away at a family reunion. Lynn described Pierre's condition: "His legs and genitals were so swollen that he couldn't point to use the urinal while lying down in bed. He'd have to sit up to pee, but he was so weak and short of breath that by the time he sat up he was gasping, his heart was pounding, and his limbs were trembling. This brought on such a panic that he couldn't pee. A few tries at this, and he was like a wet dishrag. So I said the hated word, 'diapers.' Two weeks earlier he would have died before he'd consent to wearing diapers."

Lynn put on a diaper, then whisked it off Pierre's body when it was wet. "He asked me to put another one on and leave it there," she said. "At that point he relaxed and finally slept through the night. When he woke up, he reacted like I'd discovered some medical miracle."

When I came to visit that week, Pierre seemed content, even chatty. He lay in bed, breathing from an oxygen tank, diapers under his pajamas, his legs swollen and oozing, unable to walk, the purple KS lesions now visible on almost every part of his body. Every one of these things, alone, had once been among his personal criteria: "Suicide when that happens."

"I think Pierre has changed so much emotionally and spiritually," said his hospice nurse, Clarissa. "That's been the great thing about taking care of him—to see this amazing spiritual change. And I knew he'd been suicidal. What if he had acted on it?"

A. Alvarez, one of many writers who have attempted suicide and lived to tell about it, wrote: "the only argument against suicide is life itself. You pause and attend: the heart beats in your chest; outside . . . the light moves, people are going about their business."

I sat with Pierre and no longer asked any questions about suicide. And he never mentioned it again.

• • •

Many primitive cultures have elaborate rituals to deal with the ghost of a member of the tribe who has committed suicide. If the soul leaves in desperation, the ghost lingers on in torment. In Borneo, ghosts of Dyak tribesmen who drown themselves live forever in water up to their waists; ghosts of those who poison themselves live in houses built of poisonous wood surrounded by plants that discharge horrible fumes. The Dakota Indians believe that the ghost of a suicide forever drags behind him the tree on which he hanged himself. The myth does not stop suicides. Dakotas intent on killing themselves pick the smallest tree they can find for their final act.

The common thread behind these and other taboos about suicide is the fear that the soul might leave the body before some sense of peace or completion has been achieved. The Pythagoreans of classical Greece believed that, during life, the soul is purified. If at death this purification is complete, the soul returns to the gods. If the process is incomplete or interrupted, the soul must find another body and begin the process anew. The Pythagoreans forbade suicide.

Pierre Nadeau made the initial decision to delay his suicide so that his death would be less difficult for Alexa. But the main beneficiary, it seemed, was Pierre himself. When I first met Pierre, he was living in daily torment. His ideal body had deserted him, and without it he saw no reason to go on. During the single month in which Pierre waited to kill himself, he somehow came to terms with the fading perfection of his physique. And he found an ethereal something else that would keep him alive, and content, through his increasingly severe illness.

Renee Sahm had not needed an Alexa to keep her alive. In spite of her continued talk of suicide, her desire to live required no external encouragement; she fought a dramatic battle against her illness. And when she lost this fight, Renee continued to resist her planned suicide until the last possible moment. And even then, after she took the overdose, she still breathed the next morning.

Was it a mistake for Renee to have taken the overdose? What force drove her resistance to the suicide that her reasoning mind had believed in for years? "In a man's attachment to life there is something stronger than all the ills in the world," wrote Camus in his essay "On Suicide." "The body's judgment is as good as the mind's, and the body shrinks from annihilation."

Renee, intellectually, saw no purpose in living through that final week of hallucinatory agony. Yet even after taking the massive overdose of morphine, she lived on. Perhaps it was Renee's soul that drove her to continue breathing until that next morning, in spite of the overdose. Perchance, as the Greeks thought, her soul still needed to complete its purification. Although Renee didn't believe in a spirit that would live on after she died, maybe in the depths of her coma she had discovered *something* that clamored for a natural death. Or possibly, just those very few cells at the base of the brain that control breathing were "shrinking from annihilation," not a spiritual but a purely biological battle against death, built into the system for good reason.

It might have been true that, for Renee, living out those final weeks until her natural demise would have provided something important in her transition to whatever death might bring. Even suffering, no doubt, can have meaning. Philosopher Arthur J. Dyck, in his essay entitled "An Alternative to the Ethic of Euthanasia," states that "the courage to be, as expressed in Christian and Jewish thought . . . is the courage to accept one's own life as having worth no matter what life may bring . . . because that life remains meaningful and regarded as worthy by God, regardless of what that life may be like."

Certainly Christian theologians have argued that in suffering one gains spiritually, as did Jesus on the cross. Suffering, thereby, has its own spiritual value. As far back as 1642, Sir Thomas Browne wrote, "When life is more terrible than death, it is the truest valor to live." But theologian Dr. Joseph Fletcher has reexamined this concept in terms of twentieth-century beliefs in individual freedoms: "if suffering were truly ennobling, we would be bound to withhold all anesthetics and medical relief. While some may find the last stages of terminal illness spiritually rewarding, ethicists question whether it is a person's duty to stay alive because others insist that pain is good for him."

And even in our supposedly secular modern society, "Judaic and Christian heritage is declared to be the basis for most of our laws and much of our social policy," says Dyck. Laws that now exist to forbid assistance in suicide are based in part on the philosophical and religious belief that there is value in suffering. For Pierre Nadeau this "learning through misery" undoubtedly worked. If, to avoid further anguish, Pierre had killed himself that February of 1992, his death would have been premature. No one doubted that Pierre, and Alexa, gained significantly by his living on.

The irony is that, for Pierre Nadeau, a major factor that allowed for his desire to live, to suffer on, was his awareness that assisted suicide would be available if and when he might truly need it. Had he thought that help in dying would not be within reach whenever he might ask, he likely would have killed himself in fear at the beginning of his illness. Yet Pierre was guaranteed assistance in death only because the gay community chose to disobey the laws of his state, as well as the Judeo-Christian tenets upon which they were founded.

And Renee Sahm might not have killed herself at all had she known that the option of help from her doctor was available *if* the day came that she wanted it. Renee made her own decision about the value of suffering. When Proposition 161, the bill to allow physicians to assist in suicide, was narrowly defeated in California after the Catholic Church and other religious groups mounted a four-million-dollar media campaign against it, Renee made it clear what she thought about the role of the religious beliefs of others in controlling her life. "Those right-to-lifers," she said angrily. "What kind of life do they condemn people to? Lingering for months or years suffering terrible illnesses—is that pro-life?

What right does anybody have to tell me that I should suffer through it?"

•   •   •

Chemotherapy helped to decrease the swelling in Pierre's legs. Gordon found him standing one day, trying to make the guest bed in the living room. Before Pierre had become ill, he had never offered to make this bed. Now, he collapsed while trying.

That week, Pierre decided he'd ride on his motorcycle once more before he died. He stumbled across the room with the aid of a cane, squeezed his biker boots over his swollen feet, put on leather jacket and pants, and with the help of two people climbed on the back of his motorcycle and hung on while a friend drove him around the neighborhood. I watched in awe.

Most significantly, as Lynn noted, "The anger is totally gone. I've seen Pierre throw a lot of things and kick a lot of things in his time. Now, he says to me, 'You're right there when I need you. Thank you.' From Pierre, that is amazing."

A week later, dementia set in. Pierre calmly talked to people who weren't in the room. Sensing how close he was to death, his circus friends dedicated a performance to Pierre. During a rare coherent moment, he spoke of how much he would like to attend. When the day came, Pierre got out of bed, into a wheelchair, and traveled in Gordon's van to a park across the city. He greeted his tearful circus cohorts with all the grace of the host of the day.

Back home at the end of that day, Pierre talked about the importance of two final goals: His parents were to arrive from Quebec, and it was soon to be his thirty-fourth birthday. He wanted to be alive for both events.

I came to visit Pierre a few days before his parents were due. "You look familiar," he said, and faded away. I was to have no more conversations with Pierre.

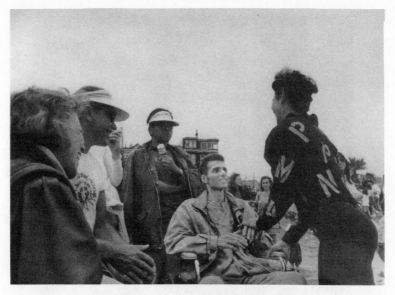

On the day his circus friends dedicated
a performance to Pierre, he met the trapeze artist
who had taken his place.

• • •

Pierre's father had been angry at his gay son before he'd acquired AIDS. The disease only affirmed his hatred of Pierre's sexuality. While Pierre remained close to his sisters and mother, his father's continued distance pained Pierre greatly.

When his parents arrived at Gordon's house the day before their son's birthday, Pierre was unconscious and clearly at death's door. His father sat on his bed, took his son's hand, told him he loved him and forgave him. He apologized for the years they had lost.

The wait began. Friends arrived, including Stephen, who had months before told Pierre he would kill him if his suffering became desperate and Pierre was incapable of doing it himself.

In the late afternoon of the day before his birthday, Pierre

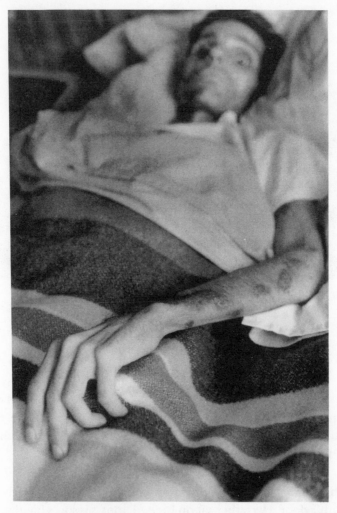

Soon after attending the circus performance,
Pierre faded from coherence.

began having seizures. His eyes rolled back, his body stiffened. Then the shaking began. He turned blue from not breathing. The first time was shocking—the family was terrified. As the day wore on the seizures increased in frequency and in ferocity. Pierre's father held Pierre down so his frail body wouldn't break, murmuring over and over through his tears, "I love you," waiting for each seizure to end.

Stephen took Pierre's parents to the living room. "When someone gets this bad," he said, "it's common to give them an overdose and end it. I have the drugs here, a gift from someone else who died of AIDS. I'm willing to do it, but it's your choice." Pierre's parents showed no surprise at Stephen's offer. They had never talked with Pierre about this, but they knew it would be what he'd want. Stephen had talked with Pierre at length; there was no question in his mind. After a short discussion, Pierre's father and mother agreed to the overdose.

It was Gordon who brought up Pierre's final goal—to live until his thirty-fourth birthday. Just past midnight, Gordon said, Pierre would achieve his last wish. Stephen would give Pierre the overdose, they all agreed, after midnight.

They waited. The seizures continued. At 9:15 P.M., Pierre stopped breathing. He rested peacefully in death.

The telephone rang. Pierre's sister was calling from Quebec, to say happy birthday to her brother. In Quebec, where Pierre had been born, it was fifteen minutes past midnight.

•   •   •

"Alexa and I never really communicated with words," Pierre had told me when I'd asked yet again about whether he had spoken to his daughter about his death.

Pierre had started making a quilt for Alexa that past Christmas. It was an image of the castle where he'd spent his Quebec childhood. "The castle burned down when I was ten," he told me. "So Alexa never got to see it. Now she'll have a quilt with my castle on it, stained-glass windows of all different colors." But he had not given it to Alexa. "There are flowers and things missing," he said. "I'll add them later."

Pierre had told no one, but during the final months of his illness he had finished the quilt. Alexa unfolded it. On the winding path leading up to the magic castle, in wondrous stitchery, Pierre had added a unicorn. From the unicorn's eye, three dark tears fell to the ground.

• • •

A few days before Pierre went into the hospital that February of 1992, five months before his death, he had asked Stephen to kill him. "It was a Saturday," Stephen recalled. "Pierre was sitting in that wing chair, and suddenly he said he wanted to do it, now. Pierre was so gorgeous and unique; everywhere he'd go he'd catch people's attention. It was all changing with his

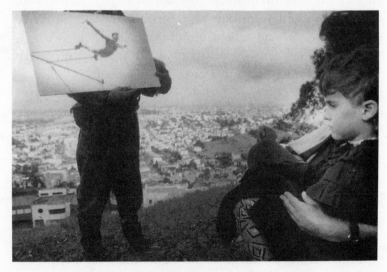

Alexa at Pierre's memorial service on a hilltop
overlooking San Francisco.

illness. But no matter what he thought, it was too soon for me to help him die."

Stephen refused to help Pierre commit suicide that day. "I'll do this for you when the time comes," he told him. "I'll commit to it, but I'm not comfortable with you just choosing to do it now."

If it does become legal for physicians to assist in suicide, many fear that the law will be abused. In spite of precautions and careful oversight, they claim that harried physicians will find it easier to encourage suicide, rather than take adequate care of dying patients; family members might have a variety of motives for encouraging someone to die; poor people who could not afford adequate care would be euthanized.

These are legitimate fears. But in my time spent with Pierre and three other gay men dying of AIDS, and with the people who had agreed to help in their suicides, I was impressed by how closely everyone followed a set of unwritten but well-understood rules—with no law in place to assure that they do so.

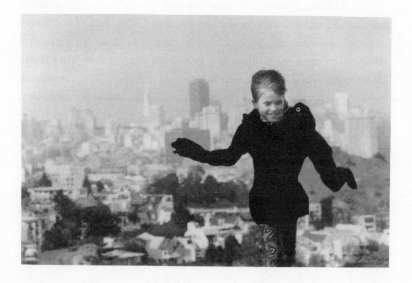

Of the four men with AIDS I grew to know, all planned to die by lethal injection. Only one actually did so. I was told dozens of stories about other people with AIDS who intended to kill themselves, yet few had carried it through. And there were many times when a request for help to die was turned down, as had happened with Pierre, because it was too soon for death. I heard of no instance that hinted at abuse.

No one knows how much abuse of assisted suicide there has been in the AIDS community, how many men and women have died prematurely because of the easy availability of lethal overdoses and of people willing to administer them. But if physicians, given the legal right to assist in hastening death, will be as careful as the gay men of the Castro seem to have been, the safeguards of close regulation and oversight should prevent almost all abuses.

And yet for the majority of people who are dying, it will be sufficient merely to know that assistance is available. They will rest assured of comfort as they progress to their natural deaths, perhaps never needing the fatal dose that is ready.

A. Alvarez, who wrote about suicide from the perspective of his own failed attempt to die, noted that "[for some] the mere idea of suicide is enough; they can continue to function efficiently, and even happily, provided they know they have their own, specially chosen means of escape always ready: a hidden cache of sleeping pills, a gun at the back of a drawer, like the wife in Lowell's poem who sleeps every night with her car key and ten dollars strapped to her thigh."

Michael White, an attorney who has studied laws for physician-assisted suicide, has concluded: "The impact of the legalization of assisted suicide is that it will extend lives—people who know that they have the *option* will live longer, and most will die smooth natural deaths while knowing that if things get too tough they have a safe and comfortable way out. But for a few, for whom natural death becomes intolerable, they will actually use assisted suicide."

Attorney White campaigned fervently for California's Proposition 161, which was narrowly defeated at the polls. I thought, along with other voters, that Prop 161 did not have the needed safeguards to become the nation's first law legalizing physician-assisted suicide.*

Yet even this loosely worded law would not have allowed for the assisted suicide of Jim Curly so soon after he received his diagnosis of cancer, as he had claimed it would in his TV commercial. Any reasonable physician, and there would have to be two according to all laws being proposed today, would have refused to assist Jim Curly in his suicide while he was so clearly depressed and not yet very ill. Pierre Nadeau and Stephen, and hundreds like them in the AIDS community, have shown the unlikeliness of Jim Curly's scenario of sudden death.

Abuses of assisted suicide do exist today. In the absence of legally available aid from physicians, abuses are occurring at the hands of unregulated freelance euthanasists, illegal suppliers meeting an otherwise unmet demand. Pierre had been dead for a year when I met Sarah, who felt she'd been placed on this earth to help others to die.

---

* In November of 1994, voters in Oregon passed a law allowing physicians to prescribe a lethal dose of medication to a terminally ill patient. But the patients must take the medications themselves; the law continues to prohibit the doctors' physical aid in the suicides. Under this law, patients who desire suicide must end their lives while still strong enough to swallow. And there is no suicide provision for suffering patients who have become too weak to take pills, nor for those who have an illness that prevents them from swallowing and keeping down an overdose.

Chapter Three

Freelance Euthanasia

———

On June 14, 1993, I sat in Gene's bedroom, watched Sarah kill him, and made no move to stop her. When I dream of that night, as I often do, I fly from the chair, seize Sarah by the arms and pull her away. I cradle Gene's unconscious body against my chest. But when I try to rouse him, Gene strikes out violently and shakes me off. Then I wake up. Even in my dreams, I never know if stopping Sarah would have kept Gene alive.

"I figured Gene and I were just going to talk about the procedure," Sarah told me months after his death, remembering her arrival at Gene's house that evening. "A bit of preparation, so to speak, to see if it's what he'd really want if things got worse. But when I got there I felt like the train was running

Author's note: Gene Robbins and Sarah are fictitious names. Certain other identifying characteristics have been omitted or obscured for reasons that will be evident to readers.

and I had to jump on." Sarah held up her hands, palms together as if in prayer; but her fingers were rigid, flesh not touching. "There was so little left inside of him," she explained, eyeing the tight space between her hands. "His loneliness, despair, the emptiness. He wanted to be gone. I got swept up in the tornado of his emotions, and I went with it; the whole nine yards."

• • •

Eugene Robbins had not been a happy man for many years, long before two strokes partially paralyzed him at the age of sixty-three. In the bedroom of his trailer home, he'd hung a portrait of Marilyn Monroe. "Believe it or not," he told me, "it's there because she looks like my wife." Gene began to sob. "She was so beautiful."

Gene's wife had been dead for eighteen years. Though he'd had scattered happy intervals since her death, his life was overwhelmed by binge drinking. And he fell in love with one married woman after another, in search of some contentment he never did find.

When he reached sixty, the burly man with the ragged white beard retired from his work as a short-order cook, took off his greasy apron, and closed up the coffee shop that had served "the best damn hamburgers in town." Then he met "Treasure," who left her husband to stay with Gene in a relationship that provided him with an upbeat interlude of two years. But when Treasure's husband became severely ill, she left Gene and went home.

Gene lay alone in bed and sliced at his wrists with a razor blade. After seventeen deep slashes, he still hadn't reached the large artery that, if sliced open, would cause him to bleed to death. Drunk and soaked in blood, he fell asleep. Gene's son found him the next morning and took him to the hospital.

Following that suicide attempt, and after some talk with

psychiatrists, Gene stopped drinking. And for one day each week Treasure left the side of her husband, whose heart was failing, to spend time with Gene. They'd go to restaurants and out dancing. He wrote her a poem.

Treasure is my valentine.
Oh, I wish that she was mine.
She will come and stay someday
when her old man goes away.
Until then we sit and wait.
That's the part that we both hate.
But not on Tuesday 'cause that's our day.
That's when Treasure comes out to play.

Gene knew Treasure's husband would soon die. Then, he hoped, she'd come live with him. But on a bus ride to a gambling weekend in Reno, his right foot suddenly felt numb. When the bus stopped and Gene tried to stand up, his leg wouldn't move. And the strength in his right arm was impaired as well. Gene's intended outing to the card tables turned into a months-long excursion to a rehabilitation hospital. He relearned how to walk, get dressed, and eat, in spite of the crippled right side of his body.

Only three months after Gene's stroke, Treasure's husband died. "He hung around," bemoaned Gene, "until I was too screwed up to be with Treasure."

After her husband's death, Treasure did want to get back with Gene. But he was too distressed by his own disease to allow it. "I was afraid that because of my stroke she'd just come for a while, then leave again," he said. "So I kicked her out."

That was the last time Gene saw Treasure, although someone kept calling him at night, hanging up when he answered. "She's checking to see if I'm still OK," thought Gene.

A few months after Treasure's departure, at four o'clock

one morning, Gene sat on the toilet, reached for the paper with his good arm, and realized he had lost the feeling in that hand as well. "I knew what was happening," he said. "I'd been through a stroke before. And there wasn't no way I was going back to the hospital." Gene stumbled about the bathroom, impulsively searching for something with which he could kill himself. Under the sink he found a variety of cleansers. He remembered the admonishment to never mix Clorox and ammonia—the combination produces lethal chlorine gas.

"I took some towels and stopped up the crack under the bathroom door," said Gene. "Then I got a bucket and dumped in the Clorox and the ammonia, set it between my legs, put a towel over my head, and inhaled the fumes."

Gene passed out. He remembers nothing until he came to on the bathroom floor. His throat burned so badly he couldn't speak. Gene crawled out of the bathroom, found the phone, and hit 911. And weeks later, when he'd recovered from the chlorine gas exposure, he looked in the phone book and called the Hemlock Society to get information about how to kill himself.

• • •

Sarah, the fifty-two-year-old president of the local county chapter of the Hemlock Society, should have gone with her first intuition when she picked up the phone and heard Gene tell his story. He emphasized that he'd had two strokes; a third could surprise him at any moment and leave him completely paralyzed, or demented. "No nursing homes for me," he told her. "I want to die before that." But Sarah heard something else behind Gene's words. "Here's a guy who's had two strokes and gives me every rational reason as to why he wants to die," she thought as she hung up the phone. "And all I can think is that I feel like playing matchmaker. This guy's just lonely."

But something about Gene intrigued Sarah. Instead of offering information, or mailing to him the usual Hemlock

Society brochures and details about lethal drugs, Sarah drove over to Gene's trailer for a personal meeting.

Gene opened the door, tilted his body so that his weak right arm swung forward, and shook hands with Sarah. "He seemed such a happy-go-lucky guy" was her first reaction. "But like he'd had a hard life thrown in there somewhere. And I liked his eyes. He had coffee heating up, and he turned out to be a jawjacker, just like me."

"When that third stroke hits," said Gene, "I'll be too far gone to kill myself, just some guy in a nursing home, throwing food over his shoulder. I've tried suicide twice." Gene didn't tell Sarah that his first attempt to take his life, the episode with the razor blade, had been a year before his first stroke. "I don't want to screw up the next time," he said.

Sarah sipped at her coffee, chatted about a variety of things, then got down to the business at hand. "That next stroke is like some sword hanging over your head," she empathized, and then explained to Gene the details of executing a successful suicide. When she got up to leave, she left a copy of *Final Exit* for Gene to read. "We've got to find a way," she said. Gene seemed puzzled. "Is this making you nervous?" asked Sarah. "Am I rushing you?"

"I think she was testing me," Gene said to me later, explaining his reaction to that first meeting with Sarah. " 'Hey,' she was telling me, 'I'm going to rattle your cage, buddy. Do you want to do it or not? Let's get with it.' " Gene paused and thought again. "She didn't really say that," he explained. "But that's the way I took it: 'If you're ready, we'll find a way. But if you're not, I'll scare you out of it.' "

Yet what most amazed Gene about this first visit with Sarah was that she offered to help with his suicide. "I don't want no one to get in trouble," he responded, puzzling out this surprising new option. "When I called Hemlock, I was just looking for information."

• • •

"Can I get personal counseling through Hemlock?" is one question addressed in the group's informational pamphlet *Q & A About Hemlock Society.* "Sorry, no" is the answer. The Hemlock Society, the booklet explains, offers only literature and information about suicide for people who have terminal illnesses, not individual guidance or physical assistance.

With a call to a local chapter of the Hemlock Society, inquirers can obtain pamphlets and books such as *Dealing Creatively with Death,* or *Final Exit.* They can subscribe to Hemlock's informational newsletter, which discusses methods of suicide, or order a "fold-out table of drugs suitable for self-deliverance, listing . . . dosages and comparative toxicity." Hemlock Society bumper stickers are also available, as are personal checks printed with the Hemlock logo, proclaiming, Good Life/Good Death. But local chapters are forbidden, by the rules of the National Hemlock Society, from offering specific advice or counseling to individuals about assistance in dying.

Yet Hemlock's local chapter leaders and volunteers speak almost jokingly about how frequently the Hemlock Society mission—one of general education about the "right to die"—is misunderstood. Desperate calls come in nearly every day from dying people and their families, saying essentially, "I'm ready now, can you come over and help?" as if Hemlock offered some home-delivery suicide service—pizzas laced with cyanide.

Each of these callers is gently advised that Hemlock does not provide suicide assistance services. Hemlock's true role, as defined by the National Hemlock Society, includes "conferences, meetings, and publications" to "educate the public about patients' rights and end-of-life issues." Though Hemlock passionately supports the right of dying people to end their own lives, and it disseminates literature describing in detail just how to do so, the society offers no specific help or individual counseling. And, certainly, Hemlock's local volunteers reject requests from individuals to come over and assist in their suicides. Or so it might seem.

In practice, the National Hemlock Society has absolutely no control over the actions of local chapter leaders and volunteers, and no method to closely monitor or even know at all what really goes on in chapters across the nation, far removed from the Oregon home office.

• • •

"From what I understand," I said to Sarah on the phone, "you're offering Gene some help in his death."

"Lonny, I am willing to sit with anybody that wants to self-deliver," she replied, choosing the favored Hemlock euphemism for suicide. "I'll talk to them, I'll hold their hands while they do it."

"What about physically assisting?" I asked.

"I would do that too," said Sarah without hesitation.

Like many people who have become deeply involved with local chapters of the Hemlock Society, Sarah's interest in the cause came from personal experience, assisting in the suicide of a loved one who suffered from a terminal illness, in Sarah's case her closest friend, Naomi. Most people withdraw after such an experience; a rare few find it to be the most significant act in their lives, and are moved to repeat it.

"To share death with somebody is incredible," said Sarah. "It's the ultimate commitment between friends."

Sarah had known Naomi for years before her friend developed a progressive disease that would destroy her nervous system. "Naomi was going to end up in a fetal position," said Sarah, "unable to move, totally dependent on everyone, without being able to talk but still able to think and understand. She looked straight at me—she had eyes like a doe—and said, 'Honey, I can't live like that.'" Long before Sarah knew anything about the Hemlock Society, or had thought about euthanasia, she clearly understood what her friend meant. "When Naomi decided to end her life," Sarah remembered, "I didn't hesitate for one second. I told her I would help."

As Naomi's illness progressed, she was confined to a hospital bed at home. Sarah spent days at a time taking care of her. One morning, Naomi asked to be dressed in her favorite nightgown. She dictated to Sarah some personal messages for her family and friends. The two sat back and watched the video *All Dogs Go to Heaven*. They drank champagne. Naomi sipped some vodka, then swallowed forty sleeping pills that Sarah had obtained for her.

Sarah held Naomi's hand and stroked her head. "You're going to go down a tunnel, hon. And at the end there's a light. And when you get there it's going to be wonderful. I guarantee it." Naomi laid her head in Sarah's lap, and she died.

"She was my idol," Sarah said years later. "My best friend, my mother. I firmly believe now that the most intimate moment you can share with a person is their death. More than sex. More than birth. More than anything. I was at the deliveries of my four grandchildren, and my experience with Naomi's death was above that."

Stephen Jamison, director of the Northern California Hemlock Society, and a Ph.D. psychologist who specializes in counseling people who are dying, knows Sarah and has thought at length about her experience with Naomi's death. "When someone reacts that positively to one encounter assisting in a suicide," said Jamison, "they'll want to do it again."

• • •

Steve Jamison sat with Gene and me in Gene's trailer home, discussing his decision for suicide. I'd already had two prior meetings with Gene and was confused by his decision to die. And I was worried about how fast things were moving with

Sarah. So I'd asked Gene if he would talk to Steve. As a counselor to the dying, Steve had vast experience in issues around suicide and illness. Steve might help Gene wade through the complex swamp of his emphatic desire for death.

Gene's wish to die was puzzling. In spite of two strokes, he seemed only minimally disabled. He was able to walk, although with the use of a cane. His right arm was weak, but he could use it for simple tasks, and his left arm worked just fine. His speech was normal. If Gene had good reason to kill himself in order to avoid the suffering of this illness, a large percentage of the elderly of our nation could just as reasonably request to die.

Gene, it appeared, had simply given up. But he elaborated a complex scheme of fear to justify his death wish: He didn't want to risk what *might* happen *if* he had another stroke.

When I mentioned to Gene the relatively good quality of life he still appeared to have, and might continue to experience for years, he responded with a well-rehearsed, one-phrase answer: "Well, whoopie shit!"

Gene planned to die, Sarah was willing to assist, and I was watching it all roll along. I wanted Steve's help to understand what was happening. And Gene clearly needed some professional aid before making his next move.

The three of us sat on stools around the counter in Gene's kitchen. While I made sandwiches, Steve talked to Gene, trying to learn the extent of his physical disability. Suddenly, Gene reached across the counter with his good arm, grabbed my right hand, and wouldn't let go. "Keep making sandwiches," he said, forcefully gripping my arm, staring at my pained expression. I dropped a piece of bread on the counter, spread mustard with my left hand, added a slice of turkey and folded the bread around it. "Now eat it," demanded Gene, pressing my now aching right hand to the counter. I picked up the sandwich and, using my left arm, raised it to my mouth. The turkey fell to the floor.

"Don't give me no more dumb shit," said Gene, "about how great my life is when I'm half paralyzed." He released my hand.

Then Gene laughed. "The fun's over," he said to Steve. "I've had it with you guys from Hemlock trying to talk me out of killing myself. I'm onto your tricks. You say you're with some organization that believes in suicide for people who are suffering. Then Sarah gets over here and tries to scare me out of it, calling my bluff, testing to see if I'll really do it. And then she sends Lonny over. We talk a few times, and it makes me feel better. Now you come"—he looked at Steve—"some fancy-pants therapist. So with all this attention I ain't so lonely. But when you leave I still can't use my arm, I'm still stumbling around with a cane, and I need some guy to lift me up and down if I want to make love to a woman. Soon I'll have another stroke and be laying around some hospital too weak to kill myself." Gene slammed his hand on the counter. "And where will you guys be then?" He stared at us. "I'm caught onto this Hemlock game," announced Gene. "It ain't going to work with me."

"Let me understand this," I interrupted. "You think that Hemlock is a group that tries to prevent sick people from killing themselves?"

"Well, they ain't what they say they are, that's for sure," replied Gene. "I know what you guys are trying to do, and it's working too. I feel better with you all stopping by, playing your games with me. But it ain't going to make no difference. I'm going to kill myself no matter what you say."

Steve put his hand on Gene's, but Gene drew away. "I'll be frank," Steve pushed on. "I've advised a lot of people about dying. And sometimes I've agreed when they've wanted to kill themselves. But from what you've told me, and what I've heard about you, you're not ready to die. And very often my role as a therapist to people who are dying—even though I work with

Hemlock—is to encourage them *not* to kill themselves. Not until they're ready. And most often not at all."

"See," said Gene, "there's the game again. But I've got your number, and it ain't going to wash with me."

"OK," said Steve, "you're right. I *am* trying to talk you out of killing yourself." He paused, sighed, and leaned back from the counter, still holding Gene's gaze. "But then I have to tell you about Sarah," he said. "Sarah was *not* kidding you. She was not testing you. When Sarah said she'd help in your suicide, she was serious. Deadly serious."

Gene stared at Steve. "You're shitting me," he said.

"Not at all," responded Steve. "Sarah got a rush from helping a friend die, and she's willing; she wants to do it again. And you need to know that, because I think it's affecting her judgment in your case."

Steve paused, his voice softened as he leaned toward Gene. "All I want to do is talk to you, to find out what you're feeling, how you've come to this desperate point." He reached again for Gene's hand.

Gene looked at me. "He does that speech pretty good, don't he?"

The sarcasm slipped by Steve. "Gene, why do you want to die?" he asked.

"I'm tired of watering the roses," replied Gene, pointing outside the trailer to the flower bed that for fifteen minutes of work each day provided his only remaining source of enjoyment in life. "There ain't nothing I can do but water the damned roses. So it's time to stop this bus and let me off."

"Gene," said Steve, rising to leave. "You need to slow this down. Think about it, talk to your family and your friends, do some homework to understand this better—it's more than just wanting to get off some bus. And damn, make some other contacts besides Sarah. If you'd like, I'm around your area every week or so. I'll stop by and we can talk. I know you think this is some con job to keep you alive—but you really do need to wait awhile before you off yourself."

"Gene," I interjected, "when I met you a few weeks ago you were ready to kill yourself right away. You said if you had the pills you'd do it that day. Now when I ask you what's going to happen, you hesitate. What's changed?"

"I'm better because of you guys, OK?" said Gene. "I'm less lonely 'cause there's folks around to talk to."

"Well, how much of your wanting to die is because you're lonely, and how much because you're afraid of the next stroke?"

Gene thought for a while. "Fifty-fifty," he concluded.

"It sounds like you're saying you're not quite ready yet," said Steve. "If you know Sarah will get you the pills, why not just wait, keep living until you really need them?"

"Last week I *was* ready to die," replied Gene. "Now I ain't so depressed or tired—so I might wait a bit." Gene saw Steve glance hopefully toward me. "But I still can't do none of the things I used to," Gene added quickly. "No hunting, no fishing. I can't be with no women. How many reasons do I have to give you guys? I ain't going to go play no bingo with the old folks. I may be lonely, like you say. But I'm also paralyzed."

"OK," said Steve. "Which of those things can you fix?"

"I know how to get out of the loneliness," said Gene. "I just don't want to. I ain't starting all over again, no matter what you tell me."

Steve and I walked from Gene's trailer to our cars. "He's so close to the edge now," said Steve, "I don't know what can keep him alive."

"I'm not sure," I replied. "He's more upbeat now than he was last week. He's talking a good story about dying, but he's having fun telling it. He's toying with us. I think something's changing."

Steve stared at the ground for a moment, then opened his

car door. "One thing's missing here," he said. "Sarah. Naomi's death was a sacred experience for her. How far will Sarah go to re-create it?"

. . .

Sarah had first learned about the Hemlock Society when Naomi became ill. She read about Hemlock in a magazine article, so when the time came to plan Naomi's suicide, Sarah looked in the phone book, found the number for her local chapter, and ordered from them the pamphlet listing lethal dosages of drugs. Then Sarah told her own physician of Naomi's plight. To her surprise, the doctor asked to see the list of Hemlock-recommended medications, then wrote a prescription for Seconal, the sleeping pill that is the drug of choice for a Hemlock-style suicide. But it was long after Naomi's death, after Sarah had climbed the ranks at Hemlock to become president of the same chapter she had first telephoned, that she realized how unusually easy it had all been.

The Hemlock Society had a rather peculiar beginning, in the love and romance columns of a British newspaper. In 1976, Derek Humphry, a journalist who wrote for the *Sunday Times* of London, placed a newspaper personal ad looking for a mate. His wife had died in 1975, and Humphry was lonely. One woman who answered Humphry's ad was Ann Wickett, an American student studying Shakespeare in London, soon to become Ann Wickett Humphry.

It was Ann Wickett who urged her husband to write down the story of his previous marriage—a deeply intimate relationship that ended when Humphry mixed a poisonous potion and, at his wife's request, fed it to her. Humphry's first wife, Jean, had been in the final stages of a painful death from bone cancer. When Ann Wickett heard the story, she was so moved that she encouraged Derek to write a book about it. *Jean's Way*, published in England in 1978, chronicled his wife's decision for suicide as her illness progressed, and Humphry's assistance in obtaining and mixing the brew of medications that "had induced prompt loss of consciousness, to be followed by peaceful death within fifty minutes."

Soon after *Jean's Way* hit the bookstores, Humphry was inundated with letters from people who were sick and wanted to know the recipe for the secret potion he had given to Jean. Also anxious to learn the details of Jean's death, and the name of the physician who supplied the medications, were the British police. In the interests of self-preservation, and the protection of his physician supplier, Humphry divulged the recipe to no one. But in response to the continued letters containing "pathetic cries for help," Humphry moved into the unenviable position of spokesman for the rights of people with terminal illnesses to have assistance in ending their lives.

Soon after the publication of *Jean's Way,* Humphry and Wickett moved to the United States, where he worked as a reporter for the *Los Angeles Times,* and continued his political drive to legalize assisted suicide. In 1980, Humphry and Wickett gathered together a group of twenty people of power whom they knew supported the legalization of euthanasia. But of the twenty, only two would publicly join them to form an organization that would advocate for the right of people with terminal illnesses to be assisted to die. "My God, they firebomb the houses of pro-abortion people," one lawyer who refused to join commented to Humphry. "What do you think they'll do to us?" Frustrated but not stopped by this low level of open support, Humphry and Wickett called a press conference to announce the formation of the new Hemlock Society, which possessed all of four members. When the press gathered about and questioned Humphry about his level of public support, he replied, prophetically, "Growing." By 1994, the National Hemlock Society boasted 72,000 members in seventy-five chapters across the United States.

But in 1980, Humphry and Wickett could not yet exhibit the bravado gained through numbers. In spite of a continuing flood of mail from people literally begging for information about how they might kill themselves, the law loomed large. Aiding someone in suicide, even if only by mailing them recipes for deadly doses, was a risky business. And Humphry was concerned about the ethics of it all. "How could I have, with good conscience," he wrote, "sent the fatal formula to people whose true medical condition I had no knowledge of?"

But as the letters kept pouring in, Humphry discovered a loophole in the law. Under the protection of the First Amendment's freedom of the press, Humphry realized he could legally publish suicide recipes intended for general public information, not specifically directed to any individual. And with that, the ethical dilemma seemed to wash away. When asked about his prior hesitancy to make deadly knowledge easily available, Humphry replied simply, "I changed my mind."

In his 1982 book, *Let Me Die Before I Wake,* Humphry placed information about lethal drugs and dosages within chatty stories about people who had taken their lives. In these accounts of real deaths, using fictitious names, Humphry described the dilemma confronted by those facing painful terminal illnesses. But as well, he included the names and dosages of the medications they used for suicide. Any savvy reader could skip the stories and philosophy and go right to the method. In this manner, Humphry began his career as the advice line to the dying.

As Hemlock continued to grow in popularity and strength, Humphry became certain that the law would not go after him for the dissemination of virtually any information to the general public. In 1991, abandoning all pretense of concealing lethal dosage information in his anecdotes of death, Humphry published *Final Exit,* a no-holds-barred description of methods of suicide that could be utilized by people who were already quite ill and weak, or by family members or friends should they decide to help out. And in one section of the book, which would later generate the most concern, Humphry described how to use a plastic bag as the only fail-safe method, in the absence of professional help, that could assure death.

The public response to *Final Exit* was stunning. A reported 520,000 Americans bought this book of recipes for suicide, putting it for eighteen weeks on the *New York Times* bestseller list, and causing a flurry of speculation: Why did half a million Americans feel the need to have an instruction manual about suicide on the shelves of their home libraries? Humphry's hunch about *Final Exit* had proven more than correct. "My journalistic antennae," he told a reporter, "told me this was going to be a big subject."

Yet somewhere along this road to success and public appeal, the ideas of Derek Humphry and his organization called Hemlock were lost. Ignored by the press, and soon, it seemed, by Humphry himself, was the fact that Humphry did not really believe people should be killing themselves at the end of an interminable illness of suffering. What he was actually fighting for was a change in the law so that physicians could legally help a patient to die. The suicide methods that motivated the sensational attention paid to *Final Exit* had nothing to do with Humphry's political platform and beliefs—that physicians should be allowed to assist in dying so that their patients' drastic attempts at suicide would become unnecessary, and families would be unburdened of the responsibility for the deaths of loved ones who were seeking help. The true Humphry/ Hemlock platform—for physician-assisted deaths—would *eliminate* the need for the suicide formulas put forth in *Final Exit.*

Final Exit, for all the attention it received, merely represented Derek Humphry's holding pattern—a frustrated response to the thousands of people who had written to him saying, "Yes, I believe the laws should be changed. But what can

I do *now?*'' So while Humphry pressed for modifications of the law, the media continued to question him about the methods of suicide advocated in *Final Exit.* It was the plastic bag, not Humphry's plea to legalize physician assistance, that became the new and famous Humphry/Hemlock symbol.

• • •

There was no doubt that Gene's change in mood—less lonely and not as obsessed with immediate suicide—had come from the sudden attentions paid to him by Steve, Sarah, and me.

But Steve and Gene were an odd pair; the intellectual, sensitive Northern California therapist was not going to connect deeply with Gene, whose most profound words about his existential angst were, "It's time to get off this bus." And Steve, in his frustration at not being able to touch Gene emotionally, had commented to me: "The only difficult choice Gene has made before this decision of whether or not to kill himself was when to flip a hamburger over for rare or well done." Clearly, these two would form no close therapeutic relationship.

Gene had virtually no significant ties in the world. His daughter and son had such tormented memories of his past attempts at suicide that he would no longer broach the subject with them. That left Sarah and me as the only two people with whom Gene was talking about his desire to die. And I had hit a dangerous dead end. As a journalist writing about suicide, if I kept in close contact with Gene, he might soon feel *obliged* to kill himself. But if I maintained my distance, Gene would sink back into his painful isolation. And it was this isolation, combined with his fear of the next stroke, that could provide the emotional thrust that would finally compel Gene to act. Gene was trapped. And I was being pulled in with him. I had no idea whether to move in closer, or to get out.

The phone woke me up late at night a week after Steve and

I had met with Gene. "He's going to die on the twenty-fourth of June," said Steve, with no other greeting.

"Who?" I moaned, half awake.

"Our buddy. It's the anniversary of his marriage to the Marilyn Monroe lady."

"When did he tell you this?" I asked.

"He didn't. Sarah just called me. They've got it all planned."

"Damn!" I said. "I intentionally haven't called him since that meeting with you. I thought we should all have some distance for a bit, Sarah included." I shook my head. "So Sarah's been there with him alone?"

"Right," said Steve, sounding unusually ill at ease. "What do we do next? I think Gene's trying to prove something to Sarah."

"Or to me," I said. "Or you." I waited. Steve said nothing. "I'll get up there tomorrow," I told him.

• • •

"What happened?" I asked Gene, again sitting at the counter in the kitchen of his trailer.

"We set a date," he announced, as if planning a garage sale.

Gene smoked one cigarette after another, alternating puffs with sips of coffee. But he was hyped beyond the effects of caffeine and nicotine. His cane scraped along the linoleum floor as he paced his kitchen, sat back down at the counter, then bounced up again. "I hope I don't blow it this time," he said.

"The last time we talked," I replied, "it seemed like you were holding off on this."

"Yeah. But I guess it's better to set a date."

"Has Sarah been up?"

"On Sunday. I told her I don't need her here. She don't have to put her neck in the noose too. It was me who brought up setting the date. June twenty-fourth is my wedding anniversary. It seemed a good date to pick."

"This is getting serious," I said.

"I've always been serious. You guys just don't get it. It ain't just loneliness. These rehabilitation exercises go nowhere. I've had two strokes in one year. How long you think it's going to be before the next one? You want me to wait around for it to happen?"

"OK, Gene," I said. "We've got three weeks to talk about it. I'll be back."

I phoned Sarah that night.

"I tried what I could," she said. "I talked to him about things he could do outside his house—join a group, go out with people, anything. I even offered to set him up with my mother." Sarah laughed. "But that next stroke—the guy's just a time bomb. No matter what I say, he wants to die. He's picked a date, and he can't do it himself." Gene had no access to deadly pills, and his paralysis prevented him from effectively using physically violent methods to end his life. "I have access to sleeping pills," said Sarah, "and we can use the plastic bag."

"Sarah," I said slowly, "you've only met with Gene three times. You barely know him."

"I like Gene," Sarah replied. "I really like him. And look what he's been through—strokes, slashing his wrists, the Clorox and ammonia thing. I couldn't stand to watch him botch it again. Look, I've been around people with mental problems. I can spot them a mile away. Gene's not that way. He's very together when he speaks to me."

I arranged to meet with Sarah and Gene on June 9, well before his selected date of the twenty-fourth. I'd wanted Steve to join us as well, but Gene refused to have him there.

"Look, I've thought about this," said Sarah after we'd set the date for our meeting with Gene. "God created me with an overwhelming empathy. I feel people's pain. Gene's feelings are now inside me. Maybe there's another way, maybe he'll change his mind. Or maybe he'll figure a way to do it himself. But if he can't, I'm going to have to decide what to do. I don't know yet."

On the night before our meeting on the ninth, Gene called me to talk about his desire to find some way to die without Sarah's help. He'd asked his doctors for sleeping pills, but because of his past suicide attempts they'd refused to give him any. And his paralyzed arm, he said, would make it impossible for him, alone, to use a plastic bag.

Gene talked about his frustration in needing someone's help with his suicide. Using a gun was out of the question. His son was still terribly upset about the bloody episode when he'd cut his wrists; Gene did not want him to live with the image of a bullet blasting his father's head apart. In fact, Gene had promised his son and daughter he would give his gun to a neighbor, to avoid any impulse to use it.

Strangely, Gene sounded almost lighthearted during our conversation. "If I could get a ride I'd go to the Golden Gate Bridge right now and try to climb over the rail," he said. "But I'd probably get hung up and everyone would think I'm some dumb Italian trying to catch an airplane." Gene giggled. "Put that in your book," he said, "then people can think that Gene was a dingleshit."

I couldn't figure out this mood. And there was something frightening about it.

"By the way," said Gene, "I don't really have to wait until the twenty-fourth, do I?" He hung up.

• • •

The meeting with Sarah and Gene the next day wasn't until 7:30 P.M. When I showed up unannounced at Gene's trailer that morning, he wasn't surprised.

"Glad you're here," he said. "I could use the company." Gene had just spent the weekend with his daughter, son, and two baby grandchildren. "They're fun," he said of the babies. "But I can't hold them anymore because I drop them. It's hard on their heads."

"You'll miss seeing them grow up," I offered.

"I won't miss them, because I don't want to miss them," said Gene, turning aside to hide the first tears he'd ever shed in my presence.

During his children's visit, Gene had given his daughter a copy of *Final Exit* to read. He didn't say why, and they didn't talk about it. When the family left, said Gene, his daughter kissed him good-bye at the door and offered her usual farewell, saying she'd see him in a month. "Honey, I'm not going to be here in a month," he told her. His daughter began to cry. According to Gene, she said nothing else.

"Do you feel like she's given her consent?" I asked.

"Yeah," replied Gene, his tears now flowing freely as he sobbed out loud. "You make me cry, damn it," he mumbled into his hands, covering his face. "I don't cry."

We sat quietly for some time. "I know how it hurt me when my mom and dad died," Gene said, breaking the silence. "And I know it's going to hurt my kids when I do."

"Does that make you think differently about your suicide?"

"No," said Gene. "But it hurts. And I can't stand the hurt of thinking about it anymore. I can't handle continuously thinking about my death until the twenty-fourth. Thinking, thinking, thinking. That's why I'm doing it today."

"Up until now, your suicide's been some distant theory," I said. "But today it's real. Is that why the tears?"

"No. My suicide's been real since I had the second stroke.

I've wanted to do it for a long time now." Gene wiped his face with his bare hand. "So why am I crying today, damn it?" He looked at me. "Am I normal?"

I remained quiet.

"Aren't you going to answer my fucking questions?" demanded Gene.

"Gene," I began hesitantly, "I can't say that wanting to kill yourself because you've had a couple of strokes is normal. I can't tell whether you want to die because you're lonely, or you're sick, or because you're afraid of getting sicker down the road."

"It ain't 'cause I'm lonely," mumbled Gene, staring down at his hands.

"When Treasure left you," I pushed on, "you slashed your wrists—a year before you had the first stroke. I'm not sure what role the strokes have played in all this."

"If not for the strokes," he replied, anger building, "I'd be sitting here with Treasure, not bullshitting with you about killing myself. I'd be out dancing, finding women. But there ain't nothing to do about that. Everybody feeds me this line about my life's not so bad—I can eat, walk, talk, all that crap."

Gene paused, staring at me across the counter. "Well, whoopie shit!" we said in chorus, and began laughing.

"See," he said, wiping at his wet eyes with the back of his hand, "now you're catching on." Gene became serious again. "Look, I'm half dead now, and it ain't going to get no better. So why go through any more? It's like getting a tooth pulled; get the son of a bitch over with."

"You have no more second thoughts?" I asked. "No hesitation, like you had last week?"

"Only when you make me cry with your fucking questions about my family," said Gene. "I've been shaking and my heart's pounding; I can't stand this suffering and thinking about it.

Shit, if Sarah can't help tonight, I'll find a way to do it anyways. Now turn off your goddamned tape recorder. I ain't talking about it no more."

• • •

At 7:00 P.M., Gene moved to his bedroom and sat on the edge of the bed, upending a bottle of vodka. He stared blindly at a TV quiz show, not bothering to turn on the sound. When Sarah breezed through the front door of the trailer, I was alone in Gene's kitchen.

Sarah, at fifty-two, had maintained a free-flowing attractiveness, with a style that most likely originated as an earth mother of the sixties, then grew into fashion sense with the New Age of the late eighties, and stopped there—a somewhat overstylized gypsy look. It fit her perfectly. Her hair was wrapped in a loose bun, strands falling across her cheeks. A bright silk scarf framed her shoulders and met the open neck of a loose brown shirt. Her long dress was held tight at her waist with an improvised silk wraparound belt. Sarah had just come from a meeting with her numerologist, she said. She was pleased with his forecast for her future.

"Gene's in the bedroom with his bottle," I told her. "He wants to do it tonight instead of the twenty-fourth." Sarah looked puzzled, then walked quickly past me into the bedroom.

Gene was sitting on the edge of the bed, facing the soundless television. The bottle of vodka was on the floor, still nearly full. His short-sleeved white shirt had popped its bottom buttons and hung open, exposing the pale skin of his protuberant belly. When he saw Sarah, Gene tried to pull his shirt together and hold it with his good hand, then gave up the effort. Sarah sat beside him on the bed, one arm around his shoulder. "Gene, are you in any condition to decide this?" she asked. He stayed silent. "What do you want to do, babe?"

Gene turned to her. "Don't ask me that," he said, without

a hint of slur to his speech. "There's a hell of a lot of things I want to do that I can't do." Gene leaned in against Sarah's body. He was flirting with her. "That's why you're here. Because there's things I can't do myself."

Sarah moved her arm from Gene's shoulder and began to massage his neck. "How do I know this is what you really want to do?" she asked.

Gene turned to me. "Go look in the fridge," he commanded. I went to the kitchen. His refrigerator was empty, and immaculately clean.

"No one's got to clean up after me," said Gene. "I threw out my food last night. And I've got my will and my casket all set. I didn't want my kids to have to do it." Gene began to sob, his chest heaving. Sarah held him tightly against her. "I won't talk about my kids." Gene's words were hard to hear through the tears, his face buried in Sarah's shoulder. "I'm so sorry I'm hurting them. But I'm going to die anyways. And I won't suffer any fucking more."

Sarah said nothing. She held Gene close with one hand, and with the other rummaged through her handbag, plucking out a pill bottle. "There's some trazodone here," she pronounced. "I took one once and it made me sleep for hours." Sarah held up the plastic container with the sedative antidepressant pills. "I think these," she told Gene, "and a bottle of vodka should do it. They'll put you to sleep, and if you don't die we can use the plastic bag." Sarah paused, then swung down and around Gene, kneeling in front of him. She lifted his downturned head so he'd meet her eyes. "If you want to do this," she said, "I'm here."

"I should do it myself," Gene responded. "I don't want to hurt anybody."

"Nobody's twisting my arm," replied Sarah.

She stood up. "I thought tonight was just the meeting to plan things," she said as she passed me on her way to the kitchen. She sighed and stopped for a moment. "But here we are."

When Sarah returned, she had Gene's "#1 Grandpa" coffee mug with her. In the bottom of the white porcelain cup was a thin watery paste, like cornstarch and water, composed of forty pulverized tablets of Sarah's trazodone, to which she'd added for good measure the contents of twenty capsules of Gene's Prozac from a container on his kitchen counter. The paste was thinned out with Lemon Zinger tea and sugar. The Prozac, an antidepressant, had been prescribed for Gene, but he never took it; he didn't think his problems could be cured by pills for depression.

"OK, toots, here you go," said Sarah, handing Gene the cup. While she was in the kitchen preparing the pills, Gene had finished a third of the bottle of vodka. He began to sip from the coffee mug. "If it's too bitter," said Sarah, "I've got some more sugar."

"Who cares if it's bitter," said Gene, swallowing the paste down.

Sarah returned to the kitchen to wash out the cup. Gene lay back on the bed, then rolled to his side. When Sarah returned, she hoisted herself alongside him and placed his head in her lap, pulling his body toward her. "Twenty years ago," said Gene, his speech beginning to slur, "I would have given you something to do on this bed."

Sarah looked down at him and smiled, her fingers stroking through his hair. "Would you have chased me?" she asked softly. Gene began to sob again, then blurted out, "I ain't going to die crying," his speech now clearly that of a drunken man. "And I ain't changing my fucking mind either."

Sarah glanced at the hand stroking Gene's head. On her wrist was a Wonder Woman watch. The busty heroine on the face of the watch, black hair flying in the wind, lasso draped over her shoulder, had clock hands centered in her bare belly. When Sarah started stroking Gene's hair, Wonder Woman's hands were at 8:10.

By 8:30, Gene had fallen asleep in Sarah's lap. She leaned over his face, her tears flowing. Gene's eyes opened briefly. "Thank you," he murmured, then began to snore.

Sarah began a quiet chant. "See the light, Gene, see the light. Go to the light, to that special place." Soon, Sarah was able to roll Gene away from her without waking him. He snored loudly.

She moved to the kitchen and returned with a large black plastic bag, into which she had put a paper towel wrapped around some ice; Humphry recommends ice to keep unbearable heat from building up inside the plastic bag. She held the ice at the top, then slipped the bag over Gene's head.

Sarah sat quietly at Gene's side, the plastic bag still loose about his neck, air flowing comfortably in. She suddenly realized, as if for the first time that night, that I was still there, sitting on the floor in the corner of the bedroom. I sat as if paralyzed, my mind racing with visions of jumping up to stop this nightmare of Gene's death.

If Sarah can't help tonight, I'll find a way to do it anyways, Gene had told me. Razor blade, chlorine gas, he'd tried twice before. *I'm going to kill myself, no matter what you guys say,* he'd shouted at me and Steve.

"Stop Sarah" raced through my mind. For whose sake, I thought—Gene's, so intent on killing himself? The weight of unanswered questions kept me glued to my corner. Was Gene's decision for death so wrong? Was this a suicide, Gene's right finally to succeed and die? Or was this a needless death encouraged by Sarah's desire to act? Had Gene's decision to have me there, to tell me his story, given me the right to stop what was happening—or, equally powerful, the responsibility not to interfere? Or was I obliged, by my very presence as a fellow human being, to jump up and stop the craziness? Was it craziness?

Events suddenly moved faster than my thoughts. Gene's body heaved up and his cry filled the room. "It's cold," he screamed, and his good hand flew up to tear off the plastic bag. Sarah's hand caught Gene's at the wrist and held it. His body thrust upwards. She pulled his arm away and lay across Gene's shoulders. Sarah rocked back and forth, pinning him down, her fingers twisting the bag to seal it tight at his neck as she repeated, "The light, Gene, go toward the light." Gene's body pushed against Sarah's. Then he stopped moving.

• • •

At midnight on June 9, three hours after Gene died, Hemlock Society's death and dying counselor Steve Jamison rolled over in his sleep and reached toward the disturbing ring coming from his phone.

"Gene's gone." It was Sarah's voice.

"Where did he go?" Steve blurted out, waking slowly.

"He's dead, Steve," said Sarah. "I helped Gene die tonight. I'm just calling to let you know that I could do this again, if I'm needed."

Steve lay back in his bed, his mind racing through the implications—for Sarah, and for the Hemlock Society—of what he had just heard.

The next day, Sarah called Steve again. "I can't get the image out of my mind," she said, "of Gene with the plastic bag over his head and me holding him down. It's haunting me."

Steve was as much astounded as he was furious. He called me right away. "Sarah is telling me this incriminating evidence over the phone," he shouted. "And it's possible that the whole organization could be held responsible. Gene found Sarah through Hemlock. She was in the role of a Hemlock representative. Not only was what she did wrong, but the whole thing could blow up and defeat this organization and its goals, and the entire movement to legitimize euthanasia." Then Steve slowed down. "I cannot get over the idea that if Gene really wanted to die," he said, "he could have found a way without criminally involving Sarah."

Steve told me he would recommend, insist, that Sarah resign her position with Hemlock. And he would somehow make her understand that unless she is as close to someone as she had been with Naomi, she could not be directly involved in a suicide. "Sarah should be giving out information that allows people to live longer and die better, not holding plastic bags over their heads while they fight to take them off," said Steve. "If Sarah refuses to resign, I will make an appearance at the next board meeting and recommend that she be removed. She's a Hemlock representative and she's out there offing people who call up to get information."

One year later, Sarah was still president of her local chapter of the Hemlock Society. No official recommendation had been made to censure her, stop her from further assistance in suicides, or even to dissolve her affiliation with the Hemlock Society. In fact, in all discussions among the leaders of the National Hemlock Society, Sarah was never referred to by her real name, only as a chapter leader in an unspecified locality. The leaders of the organization, therefore, could disavow all knowledge of her actions, purposefully evading any responsibility.

• • •

"You must *not* make housecalls," wrote Derek Humphry in frequent memos to Hemlock's local chapter leaders. "You must not get involved in other people's deaths, unless they be your own family." These injunctions had been dispatched many times during Humphry's self-described "reign of terror" as the executive director of the National Hemlock Society, which had ended in May of 1992.

Humphry had politics as much as morals in mind when he sent out this repeated admonishment to the local chapter leaders, warning against assistance in suicides. "There was a sense of self-preservation," he said, "of myself and of my organization. If there should be a lawsuit against one of our chapter leaders for assisting in a suicide, it couldn't come back to the National Hemlock Society—because we had told them they could not do this."

Yet Humphry knew specifically that there were a number of chapter leaders and other Hemlock staff members aiding in suicides. "There was a bit of elementary hypocrisy on my part," recalled Humphry, "because I knew quite well that some of the chapter leaders did it. But I would just keep my mouth shut. And if anybody questioned me, I could say, 'Here is my memo that strictly forbids this.' "

During Humphry's years at the helm of Hemlock he'd made certain that the organization was sheltered from the legal and political fallout that could descend on it from the actions of its freelance euthanasists. But because of this secrecy, no one knew how many Hemlock chapter leaders were undertaking efforts like Sarah's.

"I was first alerted to this question in 1986," said Humphry, "when an officer of the Tucson chapter helped an elderly couple to die together." The man had then told his story to the press. "My God," thought Humphry, "this is going too far! It's going to get everybody into trouble." Humphry insisted that the man be removed from his position at Hemlock. "My main problem," Humphry remembered, "was that he talked about it. I didn't mind so much him helping, but it should have been done with discretion."

And Humphry had a precedent to back up his fears. In 1980, while Humphry was in Southern California founding the

Hemlock Society, a similar organization in Britain called EXIT was heading down the tubes in the midst of scandal. Nicholas Reed, EXIT's general secretary, had been receiving phone calls from dying people, requesting information on suicide. Reed responded by sending an EXIT volunteer, sixty-eight-year-old taxi driver Mark Lyons, to their houses with a sack full of brandy, sleeping pills, and plastic bags. When Lyons' home-delivery services were discovered there were, of course, few witnesses to describe what he'd been doing. But one woman who turned down his offer to help testified that Lyons had told her, "You are the only person to disobey me."

Derek Humphry knew full well the troubles that Reed and Lyons had brought down on EXIT. Years later, Humphry took the care to write in *Final Exit*, "Actually supplying the means— drugs, plastic bag, elastic bands, etc.—may well be a crime . . . Hemlock is very careful about keeping clear of this."

Yet one leader of a chapter near Santa Barbara, California, had taken Humphry aside and said, "You know, Derek, that I go around helping people?" Humphry replied, "That's fine. Just don't tell me about it." And according to Humphry, the man "never put a foot down wrong, and went about this with complete discretion."

The self-assigned task of the National Hemlock Society is to campaign for laws that would allow physicians to assist in the suicides of people with terminal illnesses. "Hemlock's business is about changing the law, not breaking the law," said John Pridonoff, the executive director who took over after Humphry left the organization.

Pridonoff is a pastoral counselor with a doctorate in psychology and twenty-five years of experience as a therapist specializing in issues around death and dying. Pridonoff claims he is still struggling to reorganize Hemlock after Derek Humphry's departure. "This is all new territory to Hemlock," said Pridonoff, after hearing the story of Sarah and Gene.

"Hemlock as a national organization has never developed a protocol in relationship to these issues. There's nothing written in the books, as such." Pridonoff did indeed seem to be treading in unknown territory. "I don't know how often chapter leaders like Sarah are assisting," he said. "Those that involve themselves this way are private about it. They don't talk to the national office. They don't talk to me."

Pridonoff sat back and selected his words carefully. "At Hemlock, we are very concerned about chapter leaders providing *any* type of counseling. Most chapter leaders are not trained, they are not equipped to handle crisis intervention. But they *are* getting these telephone calls from desperate people, and they do not know what to do with them. While we strongly discourage our local chapter leaders from getting involved, National Hemlock has very little influence, control, or authority over the local chapters." Pridonoff spoke slowly, anxious to make his next point clear. "We are now finally in the process," claimed the executive director of the Hemlock Society, "of finding out what's really going on out there. And we do not approve of the actions of someone like Sarah."

No one at the local level who knew of Sarah's conduct ever provided her real name to Pridonoff, although the story of what occurred had reached him. Had he known about the event when it happened, and if someone had told him about it without requesting confidentiality, Pridonoff claims he would have called Sarah to say, "You can either turn yourself in, or we'll turn you in."

"That makes my blood run cold," said Derek Humphry, when advised of Pridonoff's position of turning Sarah over to the police. "If it was done with discretion," Humphry added, "I wouldn't act."

The switch-over at Hemlock, from the leadership of the charismatic but controversial Derek Humphry to the sedate, ministerial style of John Pridonoff, may indeed be a signal of change at the National Hemlock Society. Or it may not.

"In a political sense," said Pridonoff, "the name 'Hemlock' has such high visibility that we have a responsibility to maintain a level of ethical behavior. Loose cannons like Sarah can raise havoc with so much good that can come from this organization."

"Hemlock *should* be concerned about these kinds of actions," said Steve Jamison, still angry over Sarah's role in Gene's death. "But it's not because there may be a scandal. It's because people are taking actions like Sarah's all around the country."

Yet both Derek Humphry and John Pridonoff spoke almost exclusively of the potential political damage to Hemlock. Remarkably absent was any discussion of the personal tragedy of Gene Robbins, a desperate man who did not have a terminal illness, who, although at his own request, had been suffocated to death by a Hemlock chapter leader who barely knew him.

Of course, by the time Humphry and Pridonoff heard the story, Gene was dead. Nothing would change that. And it could be debated forever whether or not Gene's death was a rational voluntary suicide, a provoked suicide, or even a murder. It is no surprise that the two leaders of this large political organization reflexively moved first to protect themselves and the Hemlock Society. But it is a wonder that the prior and present leaders of the National Hemlock Society did not even pause in astonishment and dismay when they heard about what happened to Gene Robbins—and to worry greatly about how many other people who answer the telephones for the Hemlock Society continue to take such actions.

• • •

One month after Gene died, Sarah woke up suddenly in the middle of the night. "My heart was pounding, like there were earthquakes, Richter 10, going off inside me," she said. "I shook so much I wanted to crawl out of my skin." Sarah was concerned that her memories of the night with Gene were becoming too much to handle emotionally. "So I sat up and played group therapy with myself," she said. "And I still feel OK with everything that happened. But you know, I miss the guy. All I could think of that night was that I loved him."

"Sarah," I said, "you only knew Gene for a short time."

"But I really felt bonded to him," she replied. "He was so much like my father, like I'd known him forever."

Sarah's parents divorced when she was eighteen. "My father was lonely all the rest of his life," she remembered. For years, Sarah visited the house where her father lived, to fix him dinner, clean up the house. "But I knew I couldn't do anything about his loneliness," she said. "That used to just tear me up, wishing I could somehow give his life more meaning. When he died, I knew a great burden had been lifted from him."

Sarah sat quietly for a while, thinking of her father. "I've been able to take in other people's feelings since I was a child," she said. "And I could feel Gene's need, his emptiness, that big void. I loved Gene like my father. And in the end, I made him know he was loved."

• • •

Nothing, most likely, would have saved the life of Gene Robbins, who'd been intent on killing himself with or without Sarah's help. But what if Sarah had been put out of the freelance euthanasia business by some Dr. Smith down the block, acting under a new law that allowed physicians to assist in the suicides of terminally ill patients who suffered greatly at the end of their lives?

Legal scholars, medical ethicists, right-to-die organizations, and physicians who care for the dying have proposed a number of specific laws that would provide physician-assisted suicide for patients with terminal illnesses. Under virtually any of these proposed laws, Gene's Dr. Smith would have to discuss his case with another physician. Even if Dr. Smith was so moved by Gene's plight as to agree to put him to death, the second physician would point out that legal guidelines state the patient must be six months from death, according to the reasonable certainty of two physicians. And all options for treating Gene's illness and the pain associated with it must first have been tried, or at least offered.

Gene's request to die would not have passed such scrutiny. And if Gene's Dr. Smith and the second physician still agreed to put him to death, their assistance would, according to today's proposed laws, be reviewed by an "Aid-In-Dying Review Committee" and the doctors severely punished for acting outside of their allowable guidelines.

Under laws now proposing to legalize euthanasia, someone like Eugene Robbins who wanted to die would be refused any help. Gene would be right back where he started—partially paralyzed, depressed and lonely, intent on suicide, and denied help by his physicians.

And yet there would be one significant difference that might have reassured Gene: If that third stroke did arrive, and he became severely and painfully incapacitated, his wishes and beliefs were known. Dr. Smith could have reassured Gene that *if* he was badly incapacitated by another stroke, and six months from death, his stated wishes would then allow Gene's physicians to legally administer his requested lethal dose.

Even so, Gene might have killed himself. As he put it, he wanted off the bus now, not later. But possibly, if Gene's loneliness and depression had not been compounded by fear of what life would be like after a next, thoroughly incapacitating stroke, he might have withdrawn from the edge of the abyss and again found some desire to live.

At the very least, if Gene had still decided to kill himself, it would have been clear that his suicide was brought on by present unhappiness, not fear of an untenable future. And all pretenses for Sarah's assistance in his death would have been thrown to the wind.

Under a law allowing physician aid in dying, Gene might still have been a tragic and unpreventable suicide. But he would not have received an inadequate dose of a sedative medication from an untrained euthanasia specialist who alone decided to help him end his life.

• • •

It is illegal for doctors to actively help a terminally ill patient to die. But opinion polls have repeatedly shown that some two-thirds of the public favors the right of people with terminal illnesses to end their lives, and to have professional help to do it. Yet at ballot initiatives in both California in 1992 and Washington State in 1991, voters chose to continue to forbid physicians to hasten the death of dying patients who request it. And while voters in Oregon in November of 1994 passed an initiative to allow doctors to prescribe lethal doses to terminally ill patients, the law continued to forbid physicians from actively aiding in these patients' deaths. For patients too weak or ill to swallow the pills themselves, Oregon physicians still cannot legally assist in their suicides.

The difference between this majority philosophy that proclaims a belief in physician aid in dying, and the legal reality that forbids it, lies in the public's fear that the practice will be abused: Doctors might more readily help sick patients to die rather than provide them with proper (and more expensive) care; those too sick, demented, senile, or disabled to clearly articulate their wishes might be put to death without proper consent; people who are unhappy, lonely, or depressed could be inappropriately assisted or encouraged to end their lives.

Does the present illegality of physician assistance in suicide prevent such abuses, or has it merely driven the practice—abuses and all—underground?

Family members, family physicians, friends, and even freelance euthanasists like Sarah are now assisting in suicides with no more guidance than their own limited personal experiences and rules. No survey, no poll, no investigation, no educated guesses will ever yield knowledge of the number of people who have died by overdoses, plastic bags, self-inflicted gunshot wounds, or physician-administered lethal drugs—when they should instead simply have had good counseling and better medical treatment of their pain, shortness of breath, or depression.

Some significant number of assisted suicides done in hiding must fall outside of the ethical boundaries of even the most ardent supporters of euthanasia. But since the act is illegal, tales of assisted suicide are seldom told. And scrutiny of abuses is unheard of. The very illegality of the act now assures that every single assisted suicide takes place with no one monitoring it.

The present prohibition against legal assistance in suicide has guaranteed that not a single physician has ever assisted in the death of a patient while following set rules, nor under the observation of her peers, nor under the watchful eyes of the law. Yet surveys of doctors have found that up to 37 percent have, in secrecy, aided in the death of a terminally ill patient. While the public expresses fear of abuse of assisted suicide, no one is overseeing those physicians who have already made aid in suicide part of their medical practice. And certainly no one is watching the freelance euthanasists, the Sarahs, untrained and inexperienced practitioners responding to a large, otherwise unmet demand from people who are dying and are desperate for help.

The public's desire for the right to assisted suicide, with protection from abuses, is being denied on both counts. The fear of deadly abuse by physicians remains high. And rightfully so. The doctors' credo, "First do no harm," is already violated every day by poor prescribing practices and badly handled scalpels. There is no reason to assume that the practice of euthanasia by physicians will be any more perfect than the practice of medicine or surgery. But the damage that can be wrought by the surgeon's knife and the internist's prescription pad has been minimized by training, licensing, and oversight, while the damage from badly practiced euthanasia continues unchecked.

A mistrustful and worried public has every reason to deny physicians even more power over their lives—as long as they understand the uncomfortable alternative. "If legislation permitting justifiable voluntary euthanasia is not passed soon," warned Derek Humphry, "people and groups will increasingly take the law into their own hands . . . Why else would my book, *Final Exit*, sell more than half-a-million copies?"

• • •

In the quiet hours of the dawn, Renee Sahm lay unconscious yet still alive after deliberately taking a lethal overdose of morphine. And I struggled to decide whether to help her die. How easy, alone, to have made the wrong choice. At my side should have been two physicians, or an ethics review committee following the rules of a new law, to keep my personal judgment from running astray. Whatever their decision, it would have been based on principles set forth by a reasoning society, rather than the reasoning of Renee's tired and anguished friend.

"I guess I got caught up in the moment," reflected Sarah, some months after Gene's death. "And it just rolled on from there. Gene needed to be gone. And I'd like to think that if there are others like him, I'll be there for them as well."

"Sarah's going to want to feel that rush again," observed Hemlock's Steve Jamison. "For Sarah and those like her," sighed Steve, "this would be a good time to fade quietly into the background."

Chapter Four

The Slippery Slope:
Euthanasia for the Disabled

Some are proposing what is called euthanasia; at present only a proposal for killing those who are a nuisance to themselves; but soon to be applied to those who are a nuisance to other people.

—G. K. CHESTERTON

(arguing against a bill for legalized euthanasia presented to Parliament in 1935 by H. G. Wells, George Bernard Shaw, Julian Huxley, and A. A. Milne)

"I think I need much more experience in these matters of love and romance," Kelly Niles typed out on his Elkomi, a computerized communication device that allowed Kelly, with the help of an attendant, to talk. At twenty-three, Kelly was wading his way through the torture of the end of his first sexually intimate relationship. "I'm sure I'm probably pushing Debee away," typed Kelly, his spastic right hand, the one part of his body he could still control, slowly moving over the lettered keyboard as Paul, his attendant, pronounced out loud each word of the sentence. "I am full of self-pity. I'm so persistent in my attempts to make her re-love me."

Kelly Niles was indeed wallowing in self-pity, pouring word after agonizing word into what he would later call "The Debee

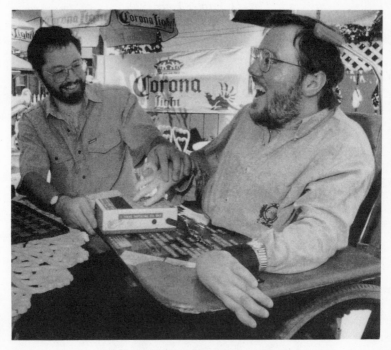

Kelly Niles with his attendant·Paul

Journals.'' The journals begin on November 30, 1982, in the Depot Cafe, a coffee shop in the upscale town of Mill Valley, California, where Kelly often lunched with the help of one of his aides. Debee, a twenty-six-year-old petite blonde with a most outgoing manner, did not look away as she passed by the young man whose misshapen limbs were strapped to his wheelchair. She paused for a moment to look curiously at the Elkomi machine balanced in front of Kelly. He wasted no time.

"Do you gotta beau?" Kelly typed out, the letters flashing one by one on the small screen of the Elkomi. They chatted for a while. Before Debee moved on, Kelly made sure to get her phone number. And after a number of dates at a San Francisco comedy club, Debee joined Kelly and his attendants on a vacation trip to Lake Tahoe, where, with the aid of one attendant, he and Debee made love for the first time.

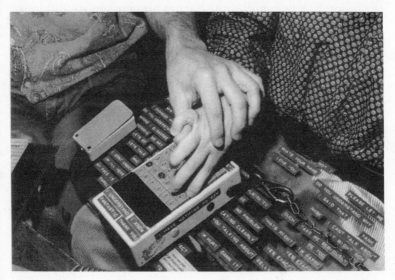

Kelly and his Elkomi.

"I have a vision today," wrote Kelly in his journal the next morning, "that nineteen-hundred-and-bloody-eighty-three will be the most painful emotional year of my life. She's my one girlfriend, first one. And as we all know, the first cut is the deepest."

That first cut of fulfilled love led to a year-long relationship with Debee—followed at its end by ten years of ever-deeper slashes brought on by the anguish of Kelly's unfulfilled longings. But not for lack of trying. After Debee and Kelly split up, he embarked upon years of bold, brazen, unarguably obsessive and often offensive attempts to find another woman. And no one, including Kelly, would argue with the fact that his failure in this endeavor was the main reason he eventually decided to kill himself.

"I feel very insecure when it comes to matters of love," wrote Kelly, during his relationship with Debee. "I need constant reassurance that Debee loves me." And yet Kelly's confusion in love came as much from his petulant youthfulness as it did from insecurity about his quadriplegia. "I see that I am a child in my lack of experience in the sexual realm," he wrote. "I feel like possessing Debee like you wouldn't believe—owning her love." When Debee, after a brief absence, told Kelly how much she had missed him, he replied, "Bullshit," and refused the hug she offered. Debee began to cry. "Why did I say that?" Kelly wrote in his journal that night. "It's just more self-pity."

Years later, when Kelly embarked on his forthright quest to die, he convinced virtually everyone he knew that self-pity had nothing to do with it. And yet Kelly was the first to admit, to emphasize, that if he could find another relationship like he'd had with Debee, he would stay alive.

Although Kelly Niles could not control his movements, his sense of taste and smell and the ability to feel someone's touch were exquisitely intact. Fine food and sex became the sensory wonders of Kelly's life. He could purchase both and often did. Kelly, his wheelchair, Elkomi, and attendants became well-known and respected visitors at some of the best restaurants in town. And Kelly formed long-term arrangements with his favorite women "masseuses."

But for Kelly, good sex, superb food, and the company of friends were not enough to drive his desire to live. "I'm getting laid tomorrow," he interjected one day in a conversation with Ram Dass about his pending suicide. The former Harvard psychologist who later gained fame as a guru immersed in meditative Eastern religions had become Kelly's spiritual advisor and grew to be a good friend. "If I could have a relationship with a woman," Kelly told Ram Dass, "I would stay around for *this* life."

"Kelly," offered Ram Dass, searching for some way to reach him and delay his suicide, "you can't get laid in heaven."

"I'll take that as a warning," Kelly laughed. "And I'll let you know from the other side." He continued on to explain how ten years of fruitlessly searching for another Debee had led him to a passionate desire to "leave this body," and to his willingness to also depart from the hordes of friends, family, and admirers who enriched his life.

"The one thing I've always wanted," Kelly told Ram Dass, "was physical intimacy with emotional involvement; to fall in love, totally. I mean, put yourself in my position."

Kelly's mother, father, therapist, spiritual advisor, lawyer, and dozens of close friends tried to do exactly that—to put themselves in Kelly's position in order to understand why he had become so obsessed with the desire to die. And it seems absurd to say that they supported Kelly in his decision to kill himself—although they eventually did—because of a death wish that came from his pining away for "a Debee." And yet Kelly Niles convinced every therapist, court-appointed reviewer, police inspector, psychologist, family member and friend that this yearning for death was a reasonable desire on the part of a mature and rational man.

Would these caring family members, friends and professionals, none of whom was disabled, have agreed to Kelly's suicide had he been able-bodied? Or was their agreement to his suicide wish a version of the commonly whispered reaction when confronted by someone's severe disability: "I'd rather be dead than live like that"?

People who are able-bodied, said Paul Longmore, Ph.D., an expert on the emotional complications of physical disabilities, assume that when a severely disabled person says he wants to be dead, "he must be acting rationally." This very assumption, claims Longmore, "is the ultimate act of oppression." Dr.

Longmore, a professor of history at Stanford University, is so severely afflicted by the paralysis of polio that he can breathe only with the help of a machine.

An able-bodied person who decides to kill himself out of yearning for a long-term relationship would be sent to psychiatrists and therapists who would fight to save him and would point out all of the things that make life worth living. They would never agree to his suicide. Yet when professionals, friends and family looked at Kelly Niles' spastically contorted body, watched him twist for agonizing moments to get out a single word on his Elkomi, and then heard that he wanted to die—they "understood."

"Kelly says he's had a pretty good life," observed his father, Dave. "But from my perspective, it's been pretty tough. Under his circumstances, I'd want to get the hell out. And that's what I've told Kelly: I understand, I sympathize, I empathize."

"I mean, let's be honest," said Kelly. "The fact that I can't ski really kills me." Kelly threw back his head in a spastic grin—a convulsion of humor that twisted the muscles of his face into a fixed, drooling smile that he could not subdue for minutes. Kelly's emotions were as spasmodic and seemingly uncontrollable as were his movements. Although in Kelly's mind the skiing joke had long been over, his body remained frozen for minutes more in the contorted smile. Then he typed out, "I figure it will be easier *over there*. I've had a truly wonderful life. It's time to go."

Kelly relied on round-the-clock attendants for his every move in the world. He could not walk, talk, clean himself, urinate, or make love without help. His disability resulted from an accident when he was eleven years old; he was thirty-three when he decided to "cross over" or "leave this body," his two favorite euphemisms for dying. But while Kelly was able to think clearly and make his wishes known, he had no capacity, alone, to cause his death.

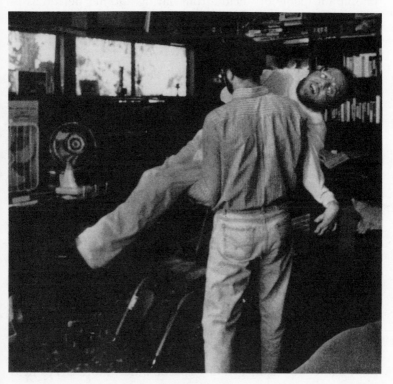

Paul and Kelly

"The ability to choose whether to commit suicide," said Andrew I. Batavia, a social worker and lawyer who is paralyzed from the neck down, "constitutes the ultimate manifestation of control over one's life. People who believe they have no control over the fundamental decision to live cannot claim to have autonomy over their lives . . . Yet we continue to prohibit people incapable of suicide from having another person assist them."

"I have the right to kill myself, like anybody else does," said Kelly Niles. "I just can't do it."

While experts debate whether laws to legalize assisted suicide might unfairly put to death people with severe disabilities, or whether disabled people have the same right to kill themselves as do the physically able, Kelly Niles struggled with his own strange personal obsession—to find a lover, or to die. For Kelly, each seemed equally impossible to achieve.

• • •

On the mantel of Joan Agnes MacMahon's study is a picture frame filled with photographs of her son, Kelly. One shot, from 1969, shows a smiling, robust ten-year-old in a Little League baseball uniform, kneeling with bat in hand, mimicking the bubble-gum-card pros. Every photo taken after that year shows Kelly with the same overwhelming smile, but the baseball uniform makes no further appearances—replaced instead in 1970 by a bulky wheelchair with Velcro straps that tied down Kelly's uncontrollably gyrating spastic limbs. More straps held the Elkomi machine that allowed the newly speechless Kelly Niles to let the rest of the world know, slowly, what he was thinking.

Over the years, what happened to Kelly at age eleven became known simply as "the accident." It took its position in a lineup of momentous family events: Kelly's parents divorced when he was six; his grandfather was buried in an avalanche when Kelly was nine; Joan Agnes' second husband, Kelly's stepfather, died from cancer when Kelly was ten.

Joan Agnes was amazed by Kelly's attitude in facing these deaths. "Why don't you talk about Grandpa anymore?" she asked him. "You were so close." "What's there to talk about?" replied Kelly. "Grandpa's OK."

Kelly's father, Dave, who shared custody with Joan Agnes, was a student of Buddhism and comparative religions. It was from Dave that Kelly received his first taste of belief in an afterlife and reincarnation. "Kelly had this remarkable attitude for the age of ten," recalled Joan Agnes, "of accepting both life and death."

Soon after the deaths of his grandfather and stepfather, Kelly Niles faced his own mortality. "There are a number of descriptions of the accident," said Joan Agnes. "Kelly likes us to say he was disabled in the Vietnam War. My God, he was only eleven! Yet people believe him because when they look at Kelly, all they can see is the wheelchair."

On the day of the accident, Kelly was playing baseball at the school recreation yard. In an argument with a friend about who was next up to bat, the boy knocked Kelly down and punched him in the head. Kelly was dazed. When he got up, he jumped on his bicycle and raced furiously for home. But his head hurt so much he abandoned his bike and walked, then stumbled, to his house. The neighbors heard his screams, but Kelly told them, "I'm all right, my dad's on the way." Indeed, Dave Niles was about to pick Kelly up to take him on a camping trip to New England.

When Dave arrived, Kelly had calmed down. They started the drive across the Golden Gate Bridge, and Kelly laid his head in his father's lap and seemed to sleep. Then Dave Niles suddenly heard "primitive, just unbelievable screams" coming from his son. He drove immediately to the hospital, where doctors reassured him that Kelly had merely sustained a concussion. The physicians did not discover that Kelly's screams of agony were caused by the pain of an expanding blood clot pushing on his brain. Dave took his son home from the hospital. Hours later, Kelly was unconscious, the brain damage already done. Although emergency neurosurgery saved his life, Kelly remained in a coma for six weeks. When he came to, he was unable to control the movements of his arms and legs. And he was mute.

No one could tell the extent of Kelly's intellectual impairment; he was clearly awake, but he could not move and was unable to speak. The specialists told Joan Agnes he should be placed in an institution. "He's coming home with me," she said. "And that's all there is to it."

Kelly received four million dollars from a malpractice suit against the doctors who had failed to diagnose the bleeding that caused his paralysis. With that money, he was able to receive years of the most advanced rehabilitation training. Kelly learned to use the spastic but slightly controllable movements of his right hand to indicate letters on the Elkomi machine. When he finally learned to spell out what he was thinking, it became clear that the accident had not affected Kelly Niles' intelligence.

"I just decided he was going to have a good life," recalled Joan Agnes of the feeling she had upon realizing her son was still intellectually with her, albeit in a less capable body. "I told Kelly over and over, year after year, that he could overcome everything, he could become whatever he wanted, and that he would lead the best life he could possibly have. I just bulldozed my way through it—the best rehab hospitals, the best attendants, all to let my son know he could have a rich and full life. And it worked—it worked!—for twenty-two good years." Joan Agnes began to cry. "But I had created some fantasy," she said softly. "It wasn't real, I made a mistake. Because Kelly eventually had to confront his disability; to discover he really *couldn't* have everything everyone else had, everything I had promised him. And when Kelly finally faced that reality . . ." Joan Agnes faded off into her own hidden passageways of memory. "What else could I have done?" she added quietly.

• • •

By the time he reached twenty-two, about the time he met Debee, Kelly had no reason to doubt he could be all his mother said. He took college courses and excelled. His ability to communicate using the Elkomi became rapid, although not as fluent as speech. But most significantly, Kelly's personality evolved into an odd combination of compassion and narcissism that drew others toward him in droves. Some part of people's attraction to Kelly, of course, came from sheer voyeurism. The young man with spastic limbs, exuberant facial expressions, and his ever-present Elkomi and attendants drew hordes of curiosity seekers. Yet Kelly was able to separate those who had a passing fascination with his singular oddity from others who were sincerely interested in what he was about. And he knew well how to play to that audience; there was something about Kelly Niles that made people want to come back for more, to try to crawl under his skin and puzzle out what it must be like to live there. He became adept at using his own mysterious self to captivate others. Kelly Niles was no disabled outcast circling the fringes of a crowded classroom, restaurant, dance hall, or brothel. Wherever he was, the light seemed always to focus on Kelly. He basked in the glow.

And knowing Kelly came with a bonus. Five full-time attendants rotated around the clock to care for him. Not only was Kelly Niles intriguing, his friendship brought along the comradery of his five attendants—each of whom had their own complexly interesting reasons for dedicating their lives to being the body and voice of Kelly Niles.

"I really liked the attendants," recalled Debee, years after she and Kelly separated. "Hanging out with Kelly was like hanging out with a whole group of friends, and they became my friends too." Kelly and his aides created a unique social vortex in which people spun toward them. Over the years, Kelly became somewhat of a celebrity in town, with a complex social calendar that swept across meetings with family, friends, attendants, professors, spiritual advisors, and, when Debee came on the scene, a lover.

Ram Dass recalled his first meeting with Kelly, at a lecture he was giving on Eastern spirituality—a discourse about Ram Dass' philosophy that "life is a curriculum, you're given a certain set of events to work with, but the issue has to do with your attachments—the question is where your thoughts are."

"There are very few people in such extreme physical states as Kelly who have come to my lectures," said Ram Dass of their first encounter. "When I met him I was aware of this incredible reaction—the feeling of 'I'm glad that's not me.' And I became absolutely fascinated by that reaction, because it stood between us. His symbolic value was so powerful that I could not meet the being that was behind it. I can usually cut through what people are as symbols, of power, wealth, or whatever. But with Kelly, I felt his *lack* of power, and then my own impatience. I just wanted to make things all right for Kelly and get on with it. Then I thought, 'There is no way to get on with it. None of us can fly, we're all trapped in these bodies.' And I started to work on my relaxing with him, to not be so distracted by his intense physical being, that feeling of powerlessness. After a while it became natural—death, life, crippledness, it's just the play of form. Kelly taught me that. And Kelly grew spiritually so fast, he was so ripe for someone to come along who wasn't feeling sorry for him—or for themselves.

"We had this great moment," recalled Ram Dass, "when Kelly asked if he could introduce me at a talk I was giving to some five hundred doctors and nurses in a lecture hall near San

Francisco. So there was Kelly on this huge stage, wheelchair, limbs contorted in all directions, head thrown back, drooling, one hand spastically moving over his Elkomi while his attendant spoke each separate word: 'Ram . . . Dass . . . says . . . We . . . are . . . not . . . our . . . bodies.' It was incredible! I broke into tears, and the audience stood up and just went wild.''

There was no doubt that it was the intellectual and personal power of Kelly Niles himself that placed him at the hub of the wheel of this extensive support system. The problem, as Joan Agnes would realize only years later, was that with all the energy directed toward Kelly, it was too easy for her son to become lost in himself. The attentions of his friends, family, and attendants centered on Kelly Niles—and his thoughts focused tightly on himself as well. After years of absorbing the glow of this attention, Kelly risked becoming some precarious black hole into which all light could enter but none could escape. And around 1990, when Kelly finally confronted the real limitations brought on by his disability, his life fell apart. The only remaining direction, it seemed, was to move further into himself, and disappear.

• • •

Paul, Kelly's closest attendant and friend, guided Kelly's hand over the Elkomi, sensing flickering movement as his fingers slid over the keys during our first interview. We were all gathered in Kelly's skylighted house in an affluent Northern California suburb. "Wxlv, Lonxj, scnrt u aswd" flashed on the screen of the Elkomi. Kelly's error rate in hitting the keys was high. After interminable moments, Paul deciphered the message and pronounced out loud Kelly's first response to my question about his desire for suicide: "Well, Lonny, since you've asked . . ."

My frustration welled up; if Kelly was to continue—letter by tormented letter—to answer my questions with broad introductory expressions like, "Well, Lonny . . ." the interview would last an eternity.

It took a short while to get Kelly's message: He will communicate using the same mannerisms with which everyone speaks. I will just have to wait.

After fourteen years as Kelly's aide, Paul could dodge the errors on the Elkomi screen, sense Kelly's intent, and give voice to his words. What read as gibberish to me became language through Paul.

But in the strange hyperspace in which Kelly surrounded himself, Paul did not exist. If I looked at Paul as he recited Kelly's words, a great cry rose up from Kelly's throat, and his spastic right hand flew repeatedly to indicate the sign pasted in front of him: I'M HERE! Within minutes of my arrival, Kelly had taught me his rules.

"I've had a truly wonderful life," Kelly commented as we settled into our conversation. "It's been twenty-two years since I was injured. I've had a ton of love and friendship. But I'm still trapped, and I'm at the end of my energy. It's time to cross over."

"Cross over" was not Kelly's euphemism for death: It was his personal reality. "Since 1973," he said, "I've known about the other side. But I have no specific vision of what it will be like when I cross over." Kelly paused, threw back his head into what started as a smile but soon became a long, drooling spasm of his face and jerking movements of his body, during which he turned blue. When the smile ended, Kelly continued his thought. "The only thing I know about the other side," he said, "is it will be better for me there."

Then, with a stunning forthrightness that I would only later come to comprehend: "Lonny, I love you. You are making me think."

"OK, Kelly," I responded, "then help me understand. From what I've been told, the reason you want to die is because you've been unable to find a lover, another Debee. I suspect it's more complex than that."

"A relationship like I had with Debee," replied Kelly, "would make me want to stay around. I have the love of my friends and parents. Yet I miss the romantic attachment. But in the end, there is no love stronger than God's—and when I cross over, I'll be closer to God's love."

Paul glanced at his watch. It was time for Kelly's daily swim. He fussed with the wheelchair, pulling off the Velcro straps that attached Kelly's limbs to the outriggings, twisting levers to make the chair recline. When Kelly was finally angled on his back in a V, like an astronaut awaiting takeoff, Paul reached down, gently lifted Kelly's body, moved out to the pool, and walked slowly down the steps. With Kelly cradled in Paul's arms, the two calmly floated across the water.

Kelly's sensual pleasures were ritualized into his everyday life. His attendants fed him, took him for swims, bathed him in hot soapy water, arranged sexual massages, drove him to the ocean at night to see the stars and hear the waves. To halt any of these activities would be the same, to Kelly, as withholding food and water.

"I'm not thinking of killing myself because I'm unhappy," declared Kelly when he and Paul finished their swim. "I am not unhappy. When I cross over, I'll be moving forward in my life. If I had a mate, that would also be moving forward. After twenty-two years like this—I'm ready to move."

"If Debee hadn't happened," I asked, "would it be easier now?"

"That's a moot point," said Kelly. "For me, this is not a question of quality of life. I love my life. It's just time to move on."

Kelly's head jerked back, and his eyes fixed on a sign on the wall he wanted me to read: BE ASSURED, YOU ARE GROWING.

"Lonny," said Kelly. "Have you ever seen anyone so happy

to die as I am? I will die while repeating my mantra: 'Christ, God, Love, Maharaj Ji. Patience.' I added patience at the end, because, for me, patience is the biggest stumbling block.''

Kelly was exhausted by his long, continuous conversation via the Elkomi.

"Patience," he said by way of ending our interview, "is for those who are certain of the outcome. I no longer have the patience to wait for another Debee. But there is no way for me to cross over—without endangering someone else who would have to help me die.'' Tears ran freely down Kelly's cheeks. Paul automatically wiped them away.

"My patience," said Kelly, "is about gone."

• • •

"Perhaps," Dave Niles told Kelly, "we could have someone come over to do a blood test." He paused, making certain he had his son's attention. "Then," he continued, "instead of taking out a few vials of blood, we would take out a few quarts."

Kelly and his dad were playing out a variation of a repeated conversation: How might Kelly be helped to die, so that police detectives and the coroner's office would not discover that someone had done it? Planning Kelly's perfect murder became the father and son's substitute for playing chess together.

"Maybe," said Kelly, "if I was already dehydrated, they wouldn't have to take out so much blood?"

"I've done some more research," said Dave. "The coroner only investigates three types of deaths: murder, accident, and suicide. So we can't have it look like any of those. It has to seem like you died of natural causes."

Kelly's physical condition made it unlikely, but possible, that he might die suddenly of "natural causes." Due to poor control of his swallowing, Kelly had accidentally choked and inhaled food twice before, leading to lung infections for which he'd been hospitalized. Kelly thought his murder could be disguised to make it appear that he had accidentally choked. But Paul, Joan Agnes and Dave all agreed that the risk of discovery using this approach was too high.

Kelly's father became the chief coconspirator in helping Kelly plan his death. "Several people," said Dave Niles, "have told me they object to what Kelly's trying to do—because they love him and are going to miss him. Well, it's going to create a shock and a void in *my* life to not have Kelly around. But that's a selfish reason to deny what he wants. I'm not going to stop him because of my needs. Since Kelly's accident, I've always promised to help him overcome the limits of his disability. And he's made it absolutely clear he wants to die. As painful as it may be for me, I'm not about to abandon him now."

"Kelly's desire to cross over is so intense," said Joan Agnes, "that we have to support him—because we love him so much. He'd asked me repeatedly, 'Do I have your support, Mom?' And I'd say, 'No, Kelly, I'm just not ready yet.' But finally, I had to say yes. That was not easy; but it was an act of motherly love."

And yet Dave, Joan Agnes, Paul and the other attendants had a line they would not cross: Though they agreed with Kelly's right to decide to die, no one was willing to put their own life in jeopardy by helping him and almost certainly being found out. "This is going to be really difficult, Kelly," said Dave. "You have no history of any deadly illnesses, and you're as tough as a damn ox. How do we figure out a way to help you get what you want and not get our own butts thrown in jail?"

In every scene they rehearsed in their minds—overdose, drowning, accidental choking, taking out too much blood—it would be clear after Kelly had died that *something* out of the ordinary had happened. And there would be an investigation. Yet for Kelly to cross over while singing his mantra, someone would have to help.

Over time, Kelly became remarkably angry, seeing this as the final insult of his disability—his inability to kill himself, as an able-bodied person might do.

But Kelly was wrong. In fact, even for those without a disability or illness, it is remarkably difficult to kill yourself.

"In suicide," wrote A. Alvarez in *The Savage God*, "there has been a technological breakthrough which has made a cheap and relatively painless death democratically available to everyone." Alvarez, however, failed to mention just what this method of suicide might be. In reality, modern technology has made today's world safer, and killing yourself a much more difficult task.

Thirty years ago, barbiturates such as Seconal (the Hemlock Society's most recommended suicide drug) were the most widely prescribed sleeping pills. If you told your doctor you needed something to help you sleep, you'd get a prescription for Seconal. Swallow the pills all at once, and you'd die. But if you walked into a doctor's office today complaining of insomnia, you'd receive one of dozens of newer drugs—Halcion, Xanax, Librium, Valium, Tranxene, Dalmane, Ativan, Serax. Hoard even five hundred of these pills and take them all at once, and you will sleep for a very long time—and then wake up. The newer sleeping pills, taking advantage of modern pharmacologic safety discoveries, have virtually no lethal dose. You cannot take enough to kill yourself.

In *Final Exit*'s recipes for suicide, Derek Humphry addresses the problem of the lack of lethality of the newer sleeping pills. If your doctor prescribes one of these, says Humphry, "Return to the doctor's office a few weeks later and complain that the drugs just do not help you sleep. Could you please have something stronger?" Humphry admits this second visit will most likely result in yet another prescription for a different brand of a safe sleeping pill. "Pay a third visit," suggests the indefatigable Humphry, and on and on, until you finally get the coveted forty-five lethal tablets of Seconal. But there is little chance that Humphry's scenario of doctor badgering will work. It is far more likely that the physician will finally become suspicious of your amazing insomnia and ask what you're really up to.

When Renee Sahm read *Final Exit*, before her brain tumor was far advanced and while she could still drive about town, she decided to follow Humphry's advice. But she didn't want to get involved in this charade with her own doctor. "I looked in the Yellow Pages," said Renee, "and purposely picked a doctor in a poor area of the city, figuring he's more used to people looking for drugs." Renee walked into the office, put down ninety dollars for the visit, and told the doctor she was having a hard time sleeping. She left with a prescription for Dalmane, a nonlethal sleeping tablet. "The whole thing was really discouraging," said Renee. "It was complicated, time consuming, and expensive. And it was not going to get me the medications I needed." Renee sighed in frustration. "How hard do I have to work to get this done?" It was this difficulty in obtaining lethal medications, as well as Renee's denial of her impending death, that had led to her lack of preparation for Plan B.

As recently as ten years ago, the most commonly prescribed pill to relieve depression was Elavil (amitriptyline). Unfortunately, Elavil was a tremendously lethal drug, handed out to people who were depressed and might want to kill themselves. Today, depression can be treated with Prozac, Zoloft, Desyrel, Triavil—remarkably safe drugs even if taken in overdose. In the days of Elavil, a depressed person's attempted suicide by overdose often led to death. Now, in the age of Prozac, an overdose most commonly causes a long nap.

Other methods of suicide are also less certain today. More homes have electric or microwave ovens, so even finding a gas oven in which to put your head may be difficult. And gas ovens, when left on, tend to cause explosions and fires that may harm others. Electric and microwave ovens, though, won't even turn on unless you can close the door after you've put your head in.

There is always the tried-and-true method of locking yourself in the garage with a hose connected to the car's exhaust to bring carbon monoxide into the driver's seat. But the environmentalists have been there first: Catalytic converters on today's cars protect urban air quality and have rendered car exhaust fumes nonlethal. Even if you own an older car, it is as likely to stall out while idling for hours as it is to poison you—or to leak carbon monoxide into the house and injure your family as well.

Other tactics are also dangerous to people around you. "Those intending to die by dropping an electric cable in their bathtubs," wrote Dr. George Mair, a retired Scottish surgeon who authored a manual on suicide for the terminally ill, "are advised to leave behind a large notice instructing no one to touch anything without first switching off the main current." Failing this, the person who finds and touches the deceased is likely to be electrocuted as well. "It is a matter of personal choice," Dr. Mair added, "as to whether some form of bathing attire is worn." Of course, if your bathroom is at all equipped with modern safety features, ground-fault breakers would prevent your own electrocution as well as that of the person who finds you in the tub.

The list of violent methods by which to commit suicide—from hangings, to guns, to jumping from buildings—is a long one; the more violent, the more likely to be effective. But as the British organization EXIT states in its book on suicide: "The body when found should look simply dead, not disgusting." Although violent means are used daily by people who want to kill themselves, these methods are hardly the answer for most patients who are hoping for a comfortable and swift death at the end of a debilitating terminal illness.

Only in the United States are guns the most common

means of suicide. Use a gun in your attempt to die, and you are five times more likely to succeed than by other methods. Yet as Derek Humphry has noted, "We know nothing about the so-called best ways to aim a gun, if there are in fact such best ways." Humphry's suspicion seems to be borne out by history.

In 1807, Meriwether Lewis—of the famed Lewis and Clark expedition that opened the Pacific Northwest—was made the governor of the Upper Louisiana Territory in reward for his exploits. Lewis, a man more suited for hunting and exploring than sitting at a desk, was miserable at the job. He set out for Washington, D.C., to talk with President Madison. But when he stopped for the night at an inn on the way, Lewis decided on suicide. He first shot himself in the head, creating a ghastly but nonfatal wound. Lewis stumbled to his feet, took gun in hand again, fired a round directly into his chest, and collapsed on the floor. Still alive the next morning, he was found crawling toward the kitchen of the inn, begging for a glass of water, saying, "I am no coward; but I am so strong, so hard to die." And Lewis, an able marksman, is joined in the history of failed gunshot suicides by, among others, Vincent van Gogh, who painted three canvases in the two days between the time he shot himself and the moment he finally died.

Of course, the technology that can be used to kill yourself has improved since the days of Meriwether Lewis and Vincent van Gogh. George Howe Colt, in his book *The Enigma of Suicide,* describes the death of "a disturbed and unhappy electronics engineer." The man "had set up a photoelectric cell in the window of his motel room. A wire from the cell ran to a device with heating elements, which he placed on his chest. Sunlight heated the elements, which in turn detonated a firecracker. The explosion of the firecracker released a firing pin which shot a round straight into his heart." No one knows if this engineer in the motel also followed the recommendation in Dr. Mair's suicide book: "Leave a short letter," suggested the

Scottish surgeon, "to thank the manager and apologize for abusing hospitality."

Suicide these days, and apparently in days past as well, is no simple task. Journalist Betty Rollin aided her mother in the difficult search for a method to die comfortably at the end of an agonizing fight against ovarian cancer. "If you're very sick," observed Rollin after her mother died, "and not prone to violence, it can be very hard to die decently." After writing a book about her experience with her mother, Rollin received hundreds of letters. "Among the saddest," she said, "are from people—or the close relatives of people—who have tried to die, failed, and suffered even more."

Dr. Neil Kessel, in an article entitled "Self-Poisoning," claimed that in the wake of the modern technological revolution in pharmaceuticals, "The way has thus been opened for self-poisoning to flourish . . . Facilities for self-poisoning have been placed within the reach of everyone." Actually, modern technology has had the opposite effect. From safer sleeping pills to air bags in cars, science has made killing yourself without professional help a tremendously difficult task—and a mission fraught with the potential for ghastly errors.

Writer Dorothy Parker perhaps had the most accurate view:

> Razors pain you;
> Rivers are damp;
> Acids stain you;
> And drugs cause cramp.
> Guns aren't lawful;
> Nooses give;
> Gas smells awful;
> You might as well live.

And yet the final choice in the Parker poem—to live—is not available to those who are suffering at the end of a terminal illness. For those people, help in dying from their physicians would be a better alternative than Parker's rivers or razors—methods also not useful to Kelly Niles, who continued his struggle to find some way to cross over.

• • •

On March 2, 1992, Kelly Niles stopped eating.

"Kelly wanted to die while still happy," said Ram Dass, "to go out singing his mantra. And it had become a fascinating problem—there was no way he could do it. But when I heard about the fast, I thought, 'Wow!'"

Yet Ram Dass echoed the concerns of others. "Personally," he told Kelly, "I don't want you to do it; I really love you and I'll miss you. Kelly, if you don't die, I'll be so happy. But, Kelly, I understand—and if you do die, I'll be so happy."

It was an earlier interchange with Ram Dass that had brought Kelly to his obsession with "going out happy." "Ram Dass told me," recalled Kelly, "that if I am attached to life at the time of death, then death would be hell. In other words, suicide should be a positive act, to move forward."

"I don't have any judgment about how a person should die," said Ram Dass in a later interview. "What the hell, it's not my business to decide what incarnation Kelly's taking." Yet Kelly had become certain that dying while happy, moving forward singing his mantra, was the route he must follow. And he designed his starvation diet to accommodate this need: "My fast will be a happy fast," said Kelly, "of water, and espressos." Espressos, Kelly added, have no nutritive value. He simply liked them.

Kelly called Debee and told her he planned to starve to death. Although it was ten years since their separation, and Debee had married and was raising two children, she and Kelly had kept in touch. When Kelly told her he planned to die, she went to see him. "I thought Kelly was only trying to get attention," recalled Debee. "He just didn't seem that dis-traught, he was still having a good time in life. I mean, here he was drinking espressos every day! I guess there was something in me that said, yes, he might continue the fast until he died. But Kelly was so extreme with me. He still had this outrageous attachment, and that would get me mad. I told Kelly I didn't want him to kill himself, but I also said, 'It's just fine if that's what you want to do.' "

Debee couldn't decide whether Kelly was simply acting to get attention, or seriously trying to die. But Debee's relationship with Kelly had ended in 1982; she had missed most of what happened to Kelly since that time.

"It was around 1990, when Kelly was thirty-one," recalled Joan Agnes, "that everything fell apart."

"We have this video of the family picnic that year," said Paul. "Everybody was having pleasant conversation, the sun was shining, flowers growing—it was really a grand scene. But there was Kelly, in the corner with me, spelling, looking tremendously sad. And I remember what he spelled: 'My life is finished.' It was the first time I realized that he was so serious."

Joan Agnes traced the change in her son to a singular incident. Kelly's favorite lunchtime hangout was Marvin Gar-dens, an upscale restaurant where one of his ex-attendants worked. "Every day," recalled Joan Agnes, "he went to this same place for lunch. He was well known there, and it was a big thing for him."

Although Kelly was unable to speak, he was not silent. When he laughed, a cry came from deep in his throat that would last for minutes. When angry or excited, or simply happy, Kelly made a variety of sounds, all loud, all long, and all poorly controlled. "Kell had lots of friends at the restaurant," recalled Paul. "They knew him well and they'd kid around with him. Kell loved it, and he'd howl with laughter." One day in 1990, a customer complained. Kelly's ex-attendant met Kelly in the parking lot at the end of the meal and asked him not to come back. "Kelly was crushed," remembered Joan Agnes. "He never once returned to that restaurant. Ever. And in my mind, that was the beginning of his social decline."

"Kelly started being sad even before that," added Paul. "Something happened when he reached thirty-one. He'd become very close to this friend, Liz, and they'd toyed for years with the possibility of having a relationship. She'd always said, 'Who knows, Kell, it may happen, it may not.' But then she finally said, 'It's not going to happen.' And something clicked in Kelly's mind; he realized he would never be married, never have children. He'd so much wanted to find a woman he could spell with, and who could lift him—so he could finally communicate with someone and be alone with her. He really cherished the idea. But after Liz, the dream died. And when he put it aside, the rest of his life didn't appear to have the excitement, the meaning, the color that had been there."

About the same time, Paul noted that Kelly was making more errors when he typed on the Elkomi. It became harder to understand him. Kelly had been through a number of custom-designed devices, one costing $35,000, each giving him the hope of easier communication. But none worked any better than the awkward Elkomi. "I think he finally realized," said Paul, "that this was the way he was going to talk for the rest of his life. And he was getting more and more frustrated with communicating; the misspellings increased. He just took a turn for the worse."

"You see," explained Joan Agnes, "I had always told Kelly, 'There is nothing wrong with your brain emotionally or intellectually—and nothing will hold you back.' I mean, we stuffed this into his head from day one. And of course he believed it! Then the restaurant, his love life, and his communication—

they all went bad. We had told him for so many years that he was capable of doing anything he wanted. And when Kelly realized it wasn't true, he took a really hard fall."

Joan Agnes, Paul and the other attendants, Kelly's therapist, Dave Niles, Ram Dass, all began to refocus, to help Kelly deal with a new view of his disability. "We became more geared toward Kelly's finally accepting his limitations," said Joan Agnes.

And Kelly became more involved in planning his death.

Kelly's mood deteriorated severely. "Got off on the wrong foot today and stayed on it all day long," says a journal entry by Kelly's aide on February 5, 1992. "Not until late tonight did the black sky break. It was the kind of day I haven't seen in Kelly for years. Today, he would not give up the despair."

Kelly's ability to assuage his loneliness through sex also seemed to end. On March 1, he prayed to "God and Maharaj Ji," asking them to "block my having sex with anyone who will leave me feeling empty and unhappy." Kelly's world seemed more and more to be closing in.

Ram Dass came by to talk. He told Kelly he'd just been to the beach, where he'd tried to ride a surfboard but couldn't catch a wave. He'd watched all the younger, stronger riders fly by. "So I just decided to enjoy the effort of *trying* to ride the wave," said Ram Dass. Then he smiled. "It didn't work," he admitted to Kelly. "But suddenly, a wave caught me and lifted me up—without my even trying." Kelly looked curiously at his spiritual advisor. "Maybe that's how you should think of your problem with women," said Ram Dass.

The next day, Kelly began his suicidal fast. "I don't believe you're doing this," one attendant said angrily. "You want love, not death." Kelly sat in tears. "You're right," he responded. "I don't know if I want to die. But I do know I want to drop this body. And I know that it will appear to you like death."

By day eight of the fast, Kelly described himself as, "Quite high emotionally, wonderfully happy about crossing over."

Although everyone agreed that Kelly had the right to choose death, all tried in every way they could to keep him from doing so. He persisted. "I love you, Mom," Kelly told Joan Agnes. "And I'm sorry I have to put you through this. But I really believe in the afterlife. And I want to go now."

On day twelve, his attendant wrote in the daily journal: "For the first time today, I feel the possibility of Kell's death. I don't want to see Kell go, but he can't stay if he himself doesn't find a reason to stay. I mean, keeping him alive against his will—Kell's powerful will!—would be outrageous. But does he really want to go?" That day, Kelly told his therapist he was "Joyfully anticipating a better life in the hereafter."

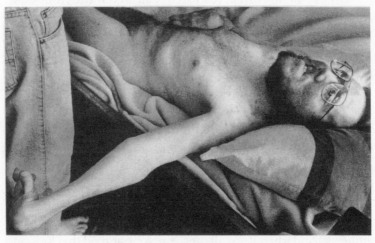

Kelly Niles

Ram Dass phoned. He was at a silent meditation retreat but broke the silence and hiked to a pay phone to talk with Kelly. "Let's not try to write the script," said Ram Dass. "Who knows? Maybe you'll walk right up to the exit, find enlightenment, then turn around and come back to share it with everyone." Kelly howled in delight. "I'm very encouraged," wrote his aide after Ram Dass' call. "The best we can do is give him love and support, and room to change his mind."

The aide had told Ram Dass they were all doing their best to support Kelly. "Which Kelly are you supporting?" asked Ram Dass. "The one who wants to live," replied the attendant immediately, then slowly added, "and the one who wants to cross over, and the one who can't bear to say good-bye, and the one who can't wait to leave—and the Kelly who just doesn't know *what* he wants to do." Kelly listened to the conversation between his aide and Ram Dass. "Why doesn't God just take me?" he asked. "This is so sad," wrote Kelly's attendant in the journal that night.

On day twenty-three, Joan Agnes answered the front door. It was the police. "I'm here to check on the welfare of Kelly Niles," said the officer, pushing his way through the door. "Well," said the flustered Joan Agnes, not quite comprehending what was happening, "Kelly Niles is *not* on welfare."

Someone had called the district attorney's office and said that Kelly's family was starving him to death, for personal gain. The police officer talked to Kelly, then filed his report. Then the social worker came, and the court investigator, followed by the sheriff. In the midst of the family crisis already surrounding Kelly's fast, the officials interviewed Kelly at length, then his attorney, his doctor and his therapist. They even called Ram Dass. Kelly, center stage, found the entire episode particularly amusing. And when it was all over, everyone agreed that Kelly was receiving the best care possible and making an independent choice. The fast continued.

On day forty-three of Kelly's fast, he began vomiting. By the next day, his pain was tremendous. "If you loved me, you'd kill me," said Kelly to anyone who approached him. No one offered. "It feels like I might be crossing over," he said, trying to ignore the pain, "and I like the possibility." But by day forty-eight, Kelly's pain from the vomiting increased, and he was too weak to even think of his mantra, let alone die while singing it. He began to eat. "To be frank," Kelly explained later, "it was just too painful to die by starvation." Kelly and his father returned once again to the now nightmarish puzzle of how Kelly Niles might end his life.

• • •

Eighteen years after David Rivlin broke his neck in a swimming accident at age twenty, he decided he'd had enough and wanted to die. Intellectually unimpaired, but so severely paralyzed he depended on a machine to be able to breathe, Rivlin petitioned the court to disconnect his respirator. The judge agreed. Turning off the breathing machine, she reasoned, would not be an illegal assistance in Rivlin's suicide, it would be the granting of his legal right to refuse medical treatment. When his doctor turned off the respirator, Rivlin quickly died.

At first glance, David Rivlin's story reads remarkably like that of Kelly Niles. But deeper in the accounts of Rivlin and Niles dwell frightening perceptions about how easily the lives and needs of people with disabilities can be dismissed: David Rivlin chose death because he lacked sufficient help to live; and Kelly Niles wanted to die, but no one could help him do it.

Kelly was thirty-three years old when he tried to starve himself to death. He had been paralyzed for twenty-two years, completely dependent on the physical assistance of others to survive. David Rivlin was thirty-eight when he decided to die. He'd been paralyzed for eighteen years. Without the aid of others, Rivlin too could not survive. Rivlin decided on suicide eight years after he and a woman named Zoe Dixon ended their one-year relationship and he gave up his dream to someday be married and have children. Kelly Niles embarked on his fast to the death ten years after the end of his relationship with Debee.

Parallel lives. But one significant difference separated Kelly

Niles from David Rivlin: four million dollars. Kelly lived at home, paid for round-the-clock attendants, bought a specially equipped van in which to travel, purchased communication equipment, attended college—all with money he'd gained from a malpractice suit against the doctors who initially failed to properly treat his head injury. Kelly Niles lived as well as his physical limitations would allow. David Rivlin received less than $300 each month from the state of Michigan, about forty-one cents per hour, to pay for the help he needed to live with his disability. Due to sheer lack of funds, Rivlin was confined to a nursing home. "If you're in a situation where you have no freedom," said Rivlin, "then you have to make a change. And my change is death."

"The case law is quite clear," Judge Hilda Gage said when she agreed with Rivlin's request to have his respirator turned off. "We are dealing with a competent adult. He has the right to refuse treatment." Gage did not mention that Rivlin might also have the right to more than forty-one-cents-an-hour's worth of assistance in dealing with his disability.

Paul Longmore, Ph.D., the disabled professor of history at Stanford University who, as Rivlin was, is dependent on a respirator, was furious about Rivlin's death. "A crippling system," said Longmore, "much more than his disability, denied Rivlin any self-determination and finally made his life unbearable." Rivlin's decision to die, asserted Longmore, was caused by "social factors—segregation, the denial of self-determination, cultural devaluation . . ." Activists around the country for the rights of the disabled looked upon Rivlin's death with horror. If Rivlin's life could be so easily dismissed, what about theirs?

"The difficulty is not in being disabled," wrote Mary Johnson, editor of the magazine *Disability Rag*. "It's in the way we treat disabled people."

"I don't want to live an empty life, lying helplessly in a

nursing home for another thirty years," said Rivlin, five days before he died. But rather than search for some way to get him out of the nursing home, the court sanctioned his death.

People with disabilities fear that judges, lawyers and physicians too easily see disabled people's lives as not worth living—and would agree to their suicides instead of working to improve their lives. Some 15,000 people with disabilities in the United States are dependent on respirators. If what happened to David Rivlin is any example, any one of these people could today be granted assistance in dying should they ask for it. Most simply need more assistance in living.

"There is this acceptance of the idea," said Michael Auberger, a quadriplegic man who heads a disability-rights project in Denver, "that it's so awful to be disabled that you would naturally want to kill yourself."

And people with disabilities are not the only large group who fear that their lives are judged to be of lesser value. Those who are simply poor worry that it will be easier to help them end their lives than to aid them in living.

"Poor people," wrote Dr. Carlos Gomez, author of *Regulating Death,* "especially in this country where we deny medical services to many of them, are the most vulnerable to be euthanized."

Would an impoverished man with cancer, confined to a crowded inner-city hospital ward, be more likely to request assisted suicide than would a man with the same disease who is living his final months at home in the company of his family, with the aid of home health-care nurses? If assisted suicide were legal, would a judge come to the side of a bedridden homeless man suffering from emphysema in a hospital ward in Harlem and quickly acknowledge his misery and grant his wish to die, while another judge might visit a man with a similar illness, well cared for at his home on Manhattan's Upper West Side, and suggest that he hang on a while longer, life is worth living?

Would a woman with health insurance who has a physician inexperienced in pain control simply switch doctors, while a woman with improperly treated pain in a crowded public hospital would instead opt for death?

In 1994, the state of Michigan formed a committee to consider legalizing physician-assisted suicide. Wilbur Howard, a black legislative lobbyist, did an "unscientific survey" in his local working-class bar, The Black and Tan, asking patrons what they thought about physician assistance in suicide. "Wilbur," they said, "we don't even trust doctors to keep us alive." Of the twenty-two members of the Michigan committee that was to decide about physician-assisted suicide, none was black. Nor were there any members who were disabled.

A report in the *Journal of the American Medical Association* in 1994 looked at care given in 297 hospitals in thirty cities around the United States. "Within each type of hospital, and even within each individual hospital," said Dr. Katherine Kahn, who headed the study, "patients from black or poor neighborhoods got less care."

At what point will this minimized care for a person who is black or poor, as it did for the quadriplegic David Rivlin, lead to a request for assisted suicide instead of a demand for better care?

Fears that the poor, minorities and disabled might be more easily encouraged to die, or will receive such inadequate health care that they would prefer to die, are well founded. But in a strange twist, the legalization of assisted suicide could actually improve health care for the poor, disabled, and minorities.

According to plans now being proposed to legalize physician aid in dying, each case of assisted suicide would be carefully regulated and monitored—at least by two independent physicians, following strict ethical guidelines, and in some proposals by an Aid-In-Dying Review Committee created specifically to evaluate every request for death. And written into a law that would legalize physician assistance in suicide could be two simple clauses: No patient would be put to death without specifically having requested it. And every patient asking to die must immediately answer one question, "Is the care you are now receiving adequate?" If the patient's answer is "No," or if the consulting physician or committee finds that control of pain, treatment of depression, or assistance in living is unacceptable—then they must first recommend better care for the patient, denying the right to suicide until all of these have been made available.

A committee that would review patients' requests to die would, in essence, become a final grievance committee, the strongest advocate for a patient's right to good care. When someone asks for death, the committee must first find out *why*. And if the answer is that the patient's misery comes from poor care during her illness, then the Aid-In-Dying Review Committee would offer better treatment, not death.

Had David Rivlin gone to such a committee with a request to end his life, they would first have evaluated the quality of help he was receiving to live with his disability—and they would have been appalled. But instead of examining the complexities of Rivlin's desire to die, a judge examined no more than the narrow question of his legal right to turn off his respirator. When she concluded he had that right, Rivlin died.

Lawrence McAfee, a quadriplegic who was also respirator dependent, was tossed from nursing home to nursing home, hospital to hospital, in a bureaucratic nightmare that would make David Rivlin's confinement to one place seem pleasant. Miserable with this existence, McAfee asked the courts for permission to turn off his respirator. But in the process of presenting his case to die, McAfee took the opportunity to make an impassioned plea about his life as the "prisoner of a bureaucracy that will pay for the warehousing of the disabled, but one that does not address or even consider the quality of our shattered lives."

The court granted McAfee's right to choose death. But before McAfee could give the order to unplug his respirator, so much attention had been drawn to his case that the bureaucracy broke: McAfee was provided full-time attendant care and moved to a group home where there was access to a bathroom and kitchen. That was enough. McAfee never pulled the plug.

A request for assisted suicide, in a well-crafted system, would mandate a final review of a patient's medical care and living circumstances. An Aid-In-Dying Review Committee would provide the ultimate check on the quality of care in life, before granting any patient's request for assistance in death. If 5 percent of patients from one nursing home were calling such a committee to ask for death, when the national average was 1 percent, the committee would be compelled to recommend an investigation of the nursing home, not the death of its patients. And if blacks in county hospitals were making requests for suicide at twice the rate as were whites in private hospitals, a red flag would be raised about the adequacy of services provided by that county hospital.

Only the most naive would think that this type of review of quality of care in itself would be enough to assure an equitable system of health care for people who are poor, or for minorities and the disabled. But it would provide one tier of evaluation that is now missing: When a patient asks for help in suicide, in every case someone would find out if there was a better alternative. Today, families who watch the suffering of a loved one may agree with (or sometimes carry out) his or her request for suicide—not having the knowledge, the expertise, or the power to first offer better care.

At the very least, a system that formally evaluated a person's life before granting their wish for death would have shown the difference between David Rivlin, who died because he was too poor to obtain proper care, and Kelly Niles, who desired to die in spite of the best everyone could offer.

And yet under today's laws, David Rivlin died by merely asking that his respirator be turned off. Kelly Niles had to find a more difficult path.

• • •

"My major disability right now," Kelly told Paul after he'd abandoned his first fast to the death, "is that I have no way to kill myself." Then Kelly became angry. His face flushed red, his head jerked back, his loud guttural cry echoed off the walls and overwhelmed the small room. "I can't do this myself," Kelly typed out furiously on the Elkomi, his anger making his rate of errors so high that Paul could barely decipher what he was saying. "You promised you would never treat me like I was disabled," Kelly told Joan Agnes when she came to his room, only to be confronted by her son's fury. "Why won't you help me die?"

If there had been any doubt about the seriousness of Kelly's intent to die during his starvation fast, there was no doubt about the profound depth of his death wish after that fast ended. No one had ever seen Kelly so continuously angry, tearful, and tremendously frustrated.

But the frustration and anger did not start immediately after Kelly's failure to fast to death. Kelly's first response at the end of his fast was one of relief and celebration. "Wow!" wrote an aide in the daily journal. "Kell is really back! He again has enough energy to think of others and get outside himself. I haven't seen so much wonderful communication in so long." When the attendants reached the last page in the journal in which they had documented Kelly's fast, it was another chance for celebration. "I can't believe we made it!" wrote one aide on the final leaf of the book. "It's a fine day—very high energy for Kell all day long. WE DID IT!"

But the emotional high after Kelly ended his fast was short lived. At first, the change seemed gradual. "Little things seem to make Kell angry," wrote one attendant at the beginning of a new volume of the daily journal. "I know I can be a real asshole at times," Kelly spelled out to the aide. "But so can you!"

"My life sucks," said Kelly when Paul arrived the next day. "That's the first time," Paul later recalled, "the only time that Kelly said something like that to me. It had always been, 'My mind is happy, it's this body I want to get rid of.' But this time, he was just so angry. It was an awesome thing to see Kelly set his sights on death with such an intensity and drive, to just go after it, like a train down the tracks."

Kelly's mood became so dark, so angry, that the attendants coined a new abbreviation to use in the daily log. "PBU," they wrote to describe many days: "Pissy, Belligerent, and Unhappy."

"Kelly's been asking again for help to cross over," said Joan Agnes. "Repeatedly. Repeatedly. He's just become so miserable with his life here—no, it's not his life here, he's miserable because he can't find a way to cross over to the next part of his life, because no one can help him. He keeps telling me, 'Mom, I'm so tired. I want to go now.' "

On July 22, 1992, only three months after the end of his first fast, Kelly stopped eating again. "Why will this new fast be any different than the last one?" I asked him. "Because this time," responded Kelly, "someone will help me. I can't believe they will let me keep suffering like this."

"On this second fast," said Paul, "he is so absolutely focused on his death, so determined, resolved. He's become obsessed with the thought that if only he can push hard enough, someone will eventually help him die."

But Kelly still lacked a plan by which someone could physically assist in his suicide without being discovered by the authorities and possibly sent to prison. "God's smiling on this fast," said Kelly on the fourth day, hoping for some divine intervention that would make it less painful than his last starvation attempt, which lasted forty-eight days.

But from the very beginning, the new fast seemed entirely different. By day five, Kelly was tremendously weak, and the dry heaves and severe stomach pains began. Most significantly, Kelly's mood hit an all-time low. Alternating with Kelly's anger was a sorrow so deep it seemed that it alone might kill him.

It was Paul who broke down first. Late one night, confronted by the agony of Kelly's painful starvation and emotional turmoil, Paul, who had been with Kelly for fourteen years, agreed to help in his suicide. They devised a plan. As Kelly approached death from starvation, Paul would feed him a lethal dose of Ativan, the sedative medication that Kelly took to decrease the jerking spasms of his paralyzed limbs. After the Ativan overdose, Kelly would still appear to have died of starvation. And if a coroner's investigation showed a high level of Ativan in his blood, Paul would explain that Kelly had become resistant to the medication and was taking higher than usual doses. When they finished working out their plan, Paul was in tears. Kelly was ecstatic. "Nothing excited Kelly," recalled Paul, "nothing energized him as much as the thought of crossing over."

Two days later, Paul changed his mind. "I just can't handle the emotional impact of doing it," he told Kelly. "I'm not at peace with it, and I fear I'll hate myself for helping in your death. I'll have to live with that for the rest of my life."

Kelly was furious. "I don't care how you feel," he told Paul. "You've deserted me." Kelly brought up every possible complaint that could be imagined. The seeming desertion of his most trusted aide and closest friend in the world was more than he could take. Kelly withdrew completely into a silence broken only by uncontrollable and unpredictable outbursts of anger. His torture knew no bounds, and the anguish of those closest to him grew to the same intensity. With this, Kelly Niles' elaborate and crucial support system collapsed.

After two fasts, and now this emotional nightmare coming from Kelly, the attendants had reached their limits. One by one, they talked with Joan Agnes about quitting. Kelly's mother panicked. "I can't hire new attendants," she cried, "it takes over a year to train them—and who would take a new job as Kelly's aide in the middle of all that's going on here? Kelly needs so much continuous care, skilled care. And I can't put my son in an institution, not now . . ."

Joan Agnes felt trapped. Arguments were breaking out among the attendants, and between them and Joan Agnes. When I arrived to see Kelly one afternoon, I waited outside for ten minutes while Paul and Joan Agnes screamed at each other. Kelly Niles' family was falling apart, and his own frequent and ghastly cries of anguish had become intolerable.

"No jail could be worse than watching my son suffer like this," burst out Joan Agnes. "I have always been able to help my child."

That night, Joan Agnes took out Kelly's copy of *Final Exit*, and began reading.

• • •

Derek Humphry was onstage at the First Unitarian Church in San Francisco. A reporter from the *New York Times* was there, as was a *Times* photographer, and TV cameras from local and national news. Humphry had decided, for the first time, to demonstrate in public the proper way to use a plastic bag to commit suicide. Playing to a packed audience, Humphry was at his charismatic best.

"This meeting is a disgrace," he began, "that we have to

gather here as lay people to teach each other how to kill ourselves. It is a disgrace to the medical profession to leave us to do this by ourselves. A physician-assisted death is extremely swift and easy and painless. When amateurs do it, it is fraught with pitfalls, difficulties, and increased suffering."

With that, Humphry selected a woman from the audience to come up to the stage and help him demonstrate what he claimed was the best guaranteed method of "self-deliverance." "Let me emphasize that taking your life takes careful preparation," said Humphry, "meticulous attention to detail. It's too easy to make a mistake. And waking up from one of these attempts is possibly the worst emotional experience one can have."

Humphry recommended a number of "experiments" to prepare for the actual event. First, some sort of sleeping pill is needed. "Over-the-counter sleep aids will suffice," claimed Humphry, "but you must first test them to see how many it takes to make you nod off." Then, a comfortable sitting position is preferred to lying down. Swallow the "sleep aids," don a painter's cotton mask to keep the bag from being sucked into your mouth, and place the bag over your head, with some rubber bands around the bottom at the level of your neck. Then hold the rubber bands and plastic bag away from your neck with your hands, allowing air to enter at the bottom. "When the sleeping pills make you nod off," said Humphry, "your fingers will let go of the rubber bands—and the bag will close tightly about the neck. Breathing will continue normally in the air-inflated bag, and death will follow about thirty minutes after the onset of sleep and the simultaneous closure of the bag."

News cameras flashed as the volunteer acted out each stage of the use of the plastic bag, and Humphry described in detail some of the finer points: the best location to place an ice bag to prevent heat accumulation and discomfort in the bag; the way

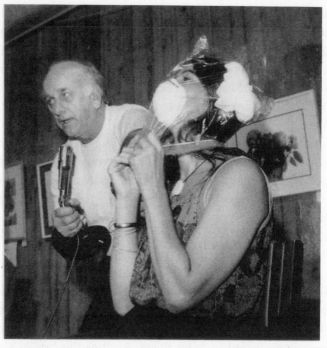

Derek Humphry onstage at the First Unitarian Church of San Francisco.

to position the fingers so as best to hold and then release the rubber bands; the aesthetic benefits of clear versus opaque plastic bags.

"Are you suffocating?" Humphry asked the volunteer, a clear plastic bag now sealed tightly about her head and neck but still inflated with air. "I'm not dead yet," she responded. "I can see that," said Humphry. "But can you breathe in there?" "Yes," the woman replied.

Humphry turned to the audience and the cameras. "She is breathing," he said. "But she is breathing poisonous air. She is in the early stages of dying." Humphry helped the woman remove the plastic bag. The audience applauded as she left the stage. "This is not suffocation or asphyxiation," announced Humphry. "It is death due to lack of oxygen."

The audience seemed puzzled. The difference between dying by suffocation or asphyxiation and "death due to lack of oxygen" appeared to elude them. In fact, no matter what the cause of death, if the person under the bag is not sufficiently sedated—either by pills or by the effect of carbon dioxide buildup in the bag—there will soon be a distressing sense of suffocation and a natural reflex to pull off the bag and suck in a deep breath of fresh air.

In spite of Humphry's recommendations, it would be remarkable if a few over-the-counter sleeping pills could bring on a slumber so deep that, when the bag finally closes about the neck, a person would not wake up in panic and fight to pull it off. Gene, with Sarah's help, had taken forty tablets of a sedative antidepressant, twenty capsules of Prozac and quite a lot of vodka. He seemed to be deeply asleep when Sarah put the plastic bag over his head—but he was soon screaming and fighting to remove it. Humphry's onstage enactment of what he claimed was a reasonable death by means of a plastic bag and a few sleeping pills seemed—if the term could be used in this context—optimistic.

I told Humphry about what happened with Gene and Sarah, wondering if he might revise his thoughts about the plastic bag. In fact, Humphry himself had never actually witnessed a plastic-bag suicide. And he'd heard many stories of failures, where people fought to remove the bag. But Humphry attributed these problems to "poor technique."

"Even without sleeping pills," said the author of *Final Exit*, "a plastic bag alone would work and be comfortable—if you're properly prepared. But the sleeping pills make it a bit more peaceful and easy." The "poor technique" used by Sarah and

Gene, claimed Humphry, was that Gene had been asleep when the bag was put on. "We all wake up a bit confused," he told me, "and Gene had had all that drink." By Humphry's analysis, Gene had awakened suddenly, been surprised to feel the plastic bag over his head, and panicked. "He should have put it on himself before he fell asleep," said Humphry. "All the failures I've heard about are from helpers jamming it on after the person is asleep. If you have to use this method, the dying person must go into it very willingly and want to carry it out—and not be surprised."

I continued to express my doubts to Derek Humphry. While we had both heard stories of plastic-bag suicides that had worked, it was difficult to believe that every failure was merely due to poor technique. And if the technique was so difficult to get right, should this really be a recommended method of suicide for people with terminal illnesses? Nonetheless, in July of 1994, Humphry sent me a copy of his new booklet describing in detail "how to perform self-deliverance using only a plastic bag and over-the-counter sleep aids." He proudly included a review from *Harper's* magazine which stated that Humphry's $5 pamphlet was a "thirteen-step plan so minutely detailed that only a fool could screw up." Humphry was pleased. "This is a breakthrough," he wrote on the copy he sent me. "The plastic bag leaflet is my new organization's bestselling piece of literature."

On November 6, 1993, the *New York Times* reported the results of a study of suicides by the New York City Medical Examiner. In that city alone, after the publication of Humphry's *Final Exit*, the number of suicides using plastic bags had increased fourfold. *Final Exit*, reported the *Times*, "has had a noticeable effect on the methods people use to kill themselves." In one-third of the plastic bag induced suicides, a copy of *Final Exit* was found at the death scene. "You could say in a disturbing way that society has benefited from the book," said

Sidney D. Rosoff, president of the Hemlock Society, to the *Times* reporter, "since there weren't as many people who had put a gun in their mouths, or who left themselves dangling from a girder on the Brooklyn Bridge." Rosoff then added his opinion that if physician assistance in suicide were legalized, "no one would have to publish self-help books." And Derek Humphry himself responded to the *Times* article, in a letter to the editor. "Three medical examiners in major American cities," wrote Humphry, "have told me privately that if they should ever need suicide to escape terminal suffering, the plastic bag would be their choice. Until we change our euthanasia laws, such self-deliverance from suffering will go on. The desperate will use anything."

• • •

Joan Agnes was desperate. She could find no way to break through the black, angry depths of Kelly's despair during his second attempt to starve to death. And Kelly's suffering was compounded by weakness from his fast, making communication with the Elkomi—his last tie to the world—an excruciating struggle. "Kell is so wasted," wrote his attendant, "that his typing hand sits as limp as a boneless cat on the tray." Nothing that his attendants, friends, or therapist could do seemed to lighten Kelly's mood, nor shift his attention to anything but death.

"So what if Kelly wants to kill himself because he's emotionally screwed up?" Joan Agnes blurted out to Paul in frustration. "We can't do anything to change it. And God, we have tried. But when it is consistent, consistent, consistent"—Kelly's mother pounded her fist on the table with each word—"is it right for him to spend the rest of his life in misery, permanently, because he cannot get help to cross over?" Joan Agnes looked straight at Paul. "It's not his anger that's getting to me," she said. "I can handle the anger. What hits me so hard is his repeatedly saying, 'If you really loved me, you'd help me, you'd have compassion. You are my mother!' "

Joan Agnes picked up Kelly's copy of *Final Exit*, walked to his room, and opened it to the section on the plastic bag. "I finally had to agree with him," she said later. "Because I loved him so much, and I have always, always been able to help him."

"Mom, I love you," said Kelly when she told him she would help him die. "I've had a good life. I am happy."

"Why not have a trial run?" suggests Derek Humphry in the plastic-bag section of *Final Exit*, to see that you can indeed be comfortable as the bag slowly brings on sedation and then death. That night, Kelly and Joan Agnes practiced with the plastic bag. Kelly was strapped into his wheelchair, head enclosed in the clear plastic, a red ribbon sealing the bag at his neck. He breathed easily and did not panic. After a few minutes, Joan Agnes removed the bag. Kelly typed out one sentence: "It will work." Then she and Kelly made plans.

First, Kelly would be given an extra dose of his Ativan sedative. When he fell asleep, Joan Agnes would place the plastic bag loosely around his head. If it woke him up, he would signal with his hand whether she should continue. And after the bag was tightened around his neck, he would signal once each minute if he wanted it to remain on. When Kelly was dead, Joan would remove the bag. A coroner's inquest would not show anything amiss; Kelly would appear to have died of his self-inflicted starvation. And if the coroner detected a higher than expected level of Ativan in his blood, it would simply be attributed to Kelly's need for a higher dose to control the increased muscle spasms brought on by the agony of his fast.

Paul called me the day after Kelly's trial run with the plastic bag. "There's a sense of lightness here with Kelly now," he said,

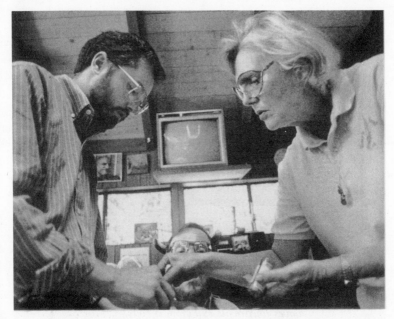

*Paul, Kelly and Joan Agnes count out Ativan pills
in anticipation of Kelly's overdose.*

"as if some weight has lifted from the air. It's so much the opposite of what's been there these past months."

It was the twenty-second day of Kelly's fast, and he was extremely weak. "I think it's the cumulative effect the two fasts have had on his already-feeble body," said Paul. "He's going downhill so quickly this time, and he's also so uncomfortable. But last week Kelly was sure he would die embittered and unhappy. Today, he's just lit up with pleasure."

Kelly arranged his death for the next day. Once the decision was made, he saw no reason to wait another moment. When Paul awakened him that morning, Kelly began his planned final day with a grand smile and a cry of bliss. They decided to spend some time together reading from *Emmanuel's Book*, Kelly's favorite volume of poetry, including a chapter entitled "Death." Paul carried Kelly to his wheelchair, placed the Elkomi by his right hand, and strapped in his other limbs. Paul began reading:

> *Even when you are dead,*
> *you are still alive.*
> *It is not a strange land you go to*
> *but a land of living reality . . .*

Kelly, so weakened by his prolonged fast, faded in and out of awareness while Paul continued.

> *If death could be seen*
> *as a beautiful clear lake,*
> *refreshing and buoyant,*
> *then when a consciousness*
> *moves toward its exit from a body,*
> *there would be that delightful plunge*
> *and it would simply swim away.*

Kelly had drifted off to sleep. Paul gently unfastened the Velcro straps that bound Kelly's limbs to the wheelchair, lifted him in his arms, and carried him to bed.

Kelly did not wake up until Joan Agnes came into the room an hour later. "Why don't you keep napping for a while," she told Kelly. "And when you wake up, I will come back and help you cross over." Kelly threw his head back and smiled. Joan Agnes bent down, lifted her son's body and held him against her. When he fell asleep in her arms, she gently lowered Kelly into the bed.

Two hours later, when Paul went to check on him, Kelly had died. Joan Agnes came into the room, saw Paul's tortured expression, then looked down at the lifeless body of her son. She and Paul stood quietly for a moment, then held each other tightly, saying nothing. Finally, Joan Agnes broke the silence. "It's what he's wanted," she said through her tears, "for so long." Paul barely got out the words. "I keep thinking," said Paul, staring at Kelly Niles, "that he's trying to move his hand—to tell us something."

• • •

"As I choose the ship in which I will sail, and the house I will inhabit, so I will choose the death by which I leave life," said the ancient Roman philosopher Seneca, who believed there could be honor in suicide. "In no matter more than in death," declared Seneca, "should we act according to our desire."

Two thousand years later, Ram Dass told Kelly Niles a somewhat more folksy version of Seneca's still-controversial idea—that we can rightfully decide to die.

"Look, Kelly," said Ram Dass, "you're given a certain set of *stuff;* everybody's got stuff. Your stuff is that you can't move and can't talk. And I've got my own problems and stuff. You're in there, and I'm in here. Interesting, no? You could work with your stuff to sainthood, use it to become a great teacher. Or you could look at your stuff and choose to die. So is your stuff an asset or a liability? I don't know. Who are we to judge?"

During the centuries that have separated Seneca from Ram Dass, some consensus has begun to emerge. We have recently entered what has been summed up as the "Rights Culture." Along with the "pursuit of happiness" and other guarantees of the U.S. Constitution, the courts have added a series of rights not specifically listed in that powerful document or its amendments: women's rights, racial rights, farmworkers' rights, prisoners' rights, tenants' rights, consumers' rights, children's rights. "In this context," says James M. Hoefler, a legal scholar and author of the book *Deathright,* "the right to die can be understood not as some ghoulish aberration, but as a natural extension of rights Americans already expect to enjoy."

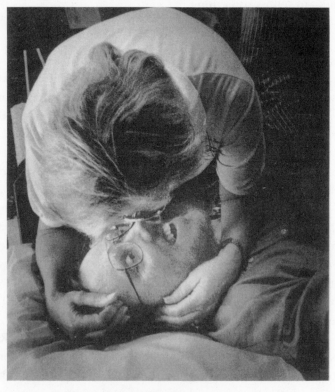

*Joan Agnes bade Kelly good night before his nap
on the day he died.*

Since there is no absolute legal, medical, or moral answer to the question of what constitutes a good or correct death in the face of a terminal illness, the power to make the decision about how someone dies can rest with only one individual—the person living in that particular body. "In the absence of an objectively valid answer, we must appeal to the individual's own preferences and values," writes medical ethicist Margaret Pabst Battin in her book *The Least Worst Death.* "Which is the greater evil," questions Battin, "death or pain? . . . it is the patient who must choose . . . To claim that an incessantly pain-racked but conscious person cannot make a rational choice in matters of life and death is to misconstrue the point: he or she, better than anyone else, can make such a choice . . ." In a televised debate about the controversy over assisted suicide, Battin fortified her stance: "I'd like to see this regarded as a profound and new civil rights issue."

But is everyone entitled to this newest aspect of the "Rights Culture," to decide for themselves when and how they should die, and to have assistance in doing it? A man who goes to his medicine cabinet and swallows the contents of a bottle of sleeping pills on the night he loses his job is not granted by society his impulsive desire for death. Rather, he can legally be dragged to a hospital, tied down, have his stomach pumped, be forced against his will to be connected to life-support machinery while he recovers from the overdose, and then committed to psychiatric care—all in the hope that his wish for death came from a temporary crisis and, with proper attention and time, he will regain his desire to live. No matter how strongly he proclaimed his "right to die" while the police or paramedics hauled him off to the hospital, his desire for death would be refused and lifesaving treatment imposed on him.

But if a man who is racked with pain, weakness, and shortness of breath in the final weeks of an inevitable death from cancer, swallowed the same overdose of sleeping pills, with the same intent to die, he could legally decline treatment, refuse to talk to a psychiatrist, and certainly reject being connected to life-support machinery that would make him survive the overdose even though he would die a few days later from his cancer. The dying man has the right to refuse medical intervention that would prolong his life; the man upset about the loss of his job is forced to accept the treatment.

Stranded somewhere between the man facing an impending painful death from cancer and the suddenly sorrowful man was Kelly Niles. Should Kelly, who had no terminal illness, have had the right to choose death and, as well, to have someone legally assist him to die? Or should the courts have intervened and committed Kelly to psychiatric care until he overcame his obsessive desire to "cross over"? If an able-bodied but unhappy adult who had no physical illness tried to kill himself, the law would demand forced psychiatric commitment and treatment until his risk of suicide diminished. Physicians and police are given every possible power to prevent such suicides. But they back off if a person is known to be terminally ill and is clear about his wish to be allowed to die. Should this same cooperation in suicide be given to people with disabilities?

Without doubt, the severity of Kelly's disability allowed friends, family, therapists, and his mother to agree that he had suffered enough in this life and could choose to leave it. But if Kelly had not been disabled, those same people would have made every possible effort to avert his self-inflicted death; and the police and court investigator who came to his house would certainly not have walked away condoning his suicide.

The boundaries become fuzzy. What if Kelly had been quadriplegic but able to speak, yet still wanted to die? Would the quadriplegia alone be enough justification for his suicide? And if Kelly's legs were paralyzed but his arms worked fine and he could get around independently in a wheelchair—what then if he still chose to die? Or if Kelly's only disability had been the need for a pair of leg braces to walk, yet he felt so badly about them he begged his mother to help him cross over—would Joan Agnes possibly have agreed?

It seemed intuitively right, when people saw Kelly's tortured body, to "understand" his wish to die. But a law that would permit a physician to assist in Kelly's death would have to draw the line at some level of disability—or it would eventually allow physicians to assist in the death of virtually anyone who claimed it was simply too difficult to go on living. Clearly, a new "civil right" granting aid in suicide would not extend to able-bodied and healthy people who were merely unhappy. But should a law that grants assistance in dying to patients who suffer from a terminal illness be extended to *all* people with disabilities?

"Equating disability with terminal illness reflects not a person's medical condition, but their devalued social status," proclaimed Paul Longmore, the disabled history professor who fears that it is too easy for people to agree with a disabled person's request for death. It is the "ignorance and bias of some nondisabled people that lead them to support such suicides," claims Longmore.

But Andrew Batavia, the quadriplegic attorney who specializes in the health rights of the disabled, disagrees. "A competent person with a disability who wishes to die," wrote Batavia, "should have the right to assistance in actively terminating his or her life . . . People with disabilities have an interest in the legalization of voluntary euthanasia even greater than that of the nondisabled population . . . After months or years of contemplating their situations, some wish to die but are unable to commit suicide without assistance . . . For those who ultimately decide that they do not want to live, we must respect that choice."

Trapped in the Longmore-Batavia debate about the rights of those like Kelly Niles to be assisted in killing themselves was Kelly Niles. The moral dilemma of whether Kelly should have been helped to die, it would seem, was only to be resolved by Kelly. "Is death the worst of harms that can befall a person," asked medical ethicist Battin, "or is unrelieved, hopeless suffering a still worse harm?" Kelly Niles had his own answer to that question, and chose death. Yet he suffered through two attempts at starvation, and his mother experienced the agony of deciding to help kill her own son, before Kelly Niles finally achieved his choice of death.

"The physician's obligation is not only to respect the patient's choices," concludes Battin, "but also to make it possible for the patient to act upon those choices. This means supplying the knowledge and equipment to enable the person to stay alive, if he or she so chooses . . . But it may also mean providing the knowledge, equipment, and help to enable the patient to die, if that is his or her choice."

• • •

Months after Kelly died, Paul and I went to see a film about Stephen Hawking, the physicist who is paralyzed, depends on a respirator to breathe, and requires a computerized voice synthesizer to speak. Hawking has perhaps come closer to understanding the physics of the origins of the universe—"as close as man has ever ventured to the mind of God"—than any human being. Admirers say Hawking achieved his "exhilarating journey to distant galaxies, black holes, and alternate dimensions" by viewing the cosmos from the perspective of his unique inner world, a spiritual place free of bodily distractions that no able-bodied person might attain. Hawking, Ram Dass might say, was using his stuff.

But while Stephen Hawking could travel the universe from the seat of his wheelchair, Kelly Niles decided he himself might get there only by dying.

And although Pierre Nadeau finally chose to live with AIDS until his last possible breath, Renee Sahm decided she'd had enough of her cancer and took an overdose, weeks before she might otherwise have died.

"Only you know how much you can take," Ram Dass had told Kelly. "So is your stuff an asset or a liability? Who are we to judge?"

Chapter Five

"Sister, Mother, Friend,
I Love You"

———

In February of 1989, fifty-six-year-old Mary Bowen Hall sat in the kitchen with Ann McGinley, her stepdaughter and closest friend. Mary had just learned that she had breast cancer and that it had already spread to her bones. "The last thing I learned from my mother," Mary told Ann, "was how to die. It was an important lesson. Now I can pass it on to you."

Ann was stunned by the news. "Couldn't you just teach me to crochet?" she responded.

Mary laughed, then got up from the table and turned away. She wanted Ann to see only the smile, not the tears that had quickly followed. A journalist and author of complex mystery novels, Mary always enjoyed the direct and straightforward manner that she and Ann shared. But on that day, Mary needed to disguise her intense fear.

"No," she said, "I'd better teach you about dying. I don't know how to crochet."

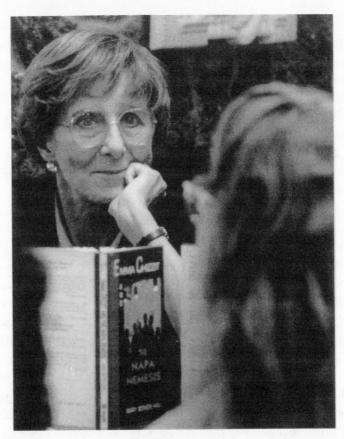

Mary Bowen Hall,
speaking at a mystery writers' conference.

Mary did think she knew about dying. "As I continue to deteriorate," she advised her forty-one-year-old stepdaughter, "it will be obscene to prop up what's left of me and have the family come take a look at it. So I've arranged to die before that."

Ann listened intently. "I've got this planned out," said the author of *The Queen Anne Killer* and *The Sacramento Stalker*. "I'll call 911. I will then lie down on the floor in the bathroom with a couple of towels under one side of my head, and I'll pull the trigger of the thirty-eight I just bought. I didn't get a twenty-two because I don't want to just do a lobotomy. I figure 911 will show up in a hurry, so my body won't lay around; and it will be professionals, not my family, who will deal with it. And in case I lose my nerve, I think I'll pull the trigger when I hear the sirens outside and they burst through the door."

Mary stared at Ann, waiting for her reaction. Her stepdaughter looked at her in disbelief. "I just want to protect the family," explained Mary Hall, "from the suffering of my death."

"Let's talk about this with your dad, and your sons" was all Ann could bring herself to say. But it was five years later, on the very day of her death, that Mary Bowen Hall would realize for the first time that she'd had it all wrong. On that final day, it was her family, especially her son Paul, who would teach Mary how to die.

And it is tempting to believe that such an unpredictable ending to her story was exactly the way Mary had planned it.

• • •

"The prospect of what's going to happen seems far off right now," said Mary when I first contacted her to see if she would talk with me about her plan for suicide. "But soon it's going to become very real. There are profound changes that will occur, in the way I'm going to see my life and in the way I'll confront death . . ." Mary paused; it was the longest she could maintain any conversation on such a serious note. Her voice shifted from the tone of the journalist and author to her preferred more folksy style. "So if you're weird enough to stick around while I go through this, well, get over here and let's have us a talk."

But our first meeting was delayed. "One of the neat things about having cancer," Mary told me when we tried to arrange an interview, "is that suddenly I've got more money than I've got time to spend it. So I just bought some plane tickets for my stepson and his family in Alaska to come down for the weekend. Why don't you come by after that?''

From the very beginning, Mary Hall's plans for death seemed filled with contradictions. She thought she might die soon and, thus, often indulged herself in "final moments," from suddenly flying family members in for a visit, to weekly pedicures at a nearby beauty salon. She even bought herself a grand "last gift" of a trip to a mystery writers' conference in London, then sailed there on the *Queen Elizabeth 2*. But while enacting these "final events," Mary also began researching and writing another mystery novel, a commitment of two or three years until its completion. And she spoke frequently about other book projects, far in the future.

There were other confusing paradoxes as well. Although she was adamant in the desire to protect her family by being alone at her moment of death, what upset them most was the thought of Mary's solitude, on the bathroom floor with a gun to her head. Mary planned to shelter the family from "those dreaded emotional farewells" she was sure would take place as she approached death. Yet some of her children felt they would need exactly the emotional final leave-taking that their mother viewed with such dread. Mary was trying to protect her family by isolating herself from them—which was the very thing that upset them the most.

Mary Bowen Hall, a writer who could neatly tie together the most convoluted twists and turns of her mystery novels, was having an impossible time plotting out the mysterious process of her own final days and her death. The scene she had outlined just didn't seem to come together into something that would work.

• • •

"I think I'm in a heap of trouble," declared Mary Hall when the cancer specialist told her, in 1989, that the most she could hope for was "remission."

"I had thought I was in the afternoon of my life, the sun shining over my shoulder," Mary conceded. "But suddenly it was a couple of minutes before midnight, and straight ahead of me was this dark shadow. I remember thinking, I'd better make some plans." Five years later, Mary was still alive, and still trying to work out the best design for her impending death.

"I've always been a terribly pragmatic person," she asserted, failing to mention the strong mischievous side that filled her life as much with jest as pragmatics. It was this combined playfulness and pragmatism that had kept her going through five years of one different cancer treatment after another, each buying her a bit more time. In one of these desperate attempts to stay alive, Mary spent six weeks in a hospital isolation room to undergo a bone-marrow transplant. Her doctors sent in a psychiatrist because she did nothing all day but lie in bed, staring at the ceiling. "Why won't you even turn on the TV?" they asked her. "How are you going to get through this time?"

"I was sorely tempted to tell them what I was doing," Mary laughed. "But it was more fun not to. So I just kept staring at the ceiling. I was laying there having a great time, thinking up murders, working out in my head a particular story I hadn't been able to write before. And it really got exciting. I created a lovely villain while I lay there waiting for my bone marrow to recover. In fact, thinking through my mysteries has enabled me to get through some of the worst times. So I just looked sternly at the psychiatrist, told him to leave, and went on with my fun."

Yet Mary never lost sight of the fact that at the end of the good she believed she could extract from the worst of times was her death. "Now that's a heck of a thing to cope with," she proclaimed. "But being dead is not going to be the problem.

It's the period just before that, when I'm barely a shell of myself, that I've still got to figure out."

• • •

On our first meeting, Mary took me for a hike on a wooded, steep hill in Annendale, a state park near her home, and her favorite place for a walk and a chat. My dog, Rosie, trotted briskly at our side. Mary's cancer, in remission at the time of our hike, had previously damaged her hip and the bones of her spine. She walked hunched over from the effects of two collapsed, cancer-invaded vertebrae, and she favored one painful hip as she climbed the hill. Yet she kept up a quick pace on the uphill stretches. "Doing this hike," said Mary, "is my way of testing myself, a way to find out how well I'm doing." She climbed rapidly up the hill. "This month," she said, "I'm doing just fine."

Before we'd gone very far, my dog disappeared. "It happens all the time," I told Mary. "She'll find her way back." But in spite of my repeated reassurances, Mary became very agitated. "That attitude you have," she said harshly, "is typical of people who are healthy. I have learned that if you want things to work out, you do something to make it happen."

I suggested that we go on with our walk, the dog would find me, she always did. But Mary went tromping off the path, up into the woods, in search of Rosie. And she didn't calm down until she'd found the dog. "She may have come back to us anyway," Mary chided me, "but if you want to be sure about things, go after them yourself."

"I wonder," I said, ready to move past Mary's lecture on the dog, "about your decision to shoot yourself. You're the first person with a terminal illness I've talked with who has decided to end her life with a gun—and to die alone, away from all the people she loves. What is going on?"

"You can't count on pills to kill yourself," Mary replied.

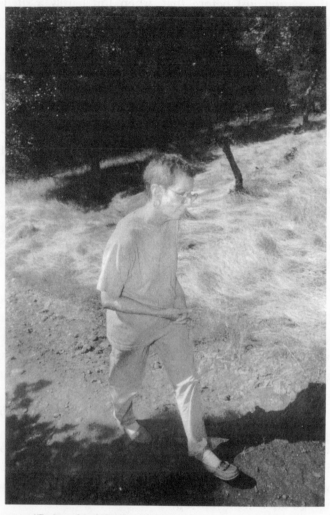

"Doing this hike," said Mary, "is my way of testing myself, a way to find out how well I'm doing."

"And that thing in *Final Exit*—take some pills, and when you're about to go unconscious, pull a plastic bag over your head. Well, I know what I can and can't do—and sitting with a plastic bag over my head, waiting to die, that's not for me. But one moment of pulling a trigger, I can handle that. It's just a pragmatic choice," she claimed, "the only suicide that will work, since I insist on being alone when I do it."

"Most people who are very ill accept some help from people who care about them," I offered, "especially when they are sick enough to be near death. 'That's what families are for,' is the expression. And yet you insist that even in your upcoming sickness, and in your death, you're protecting your family by keeping your distance. I have to wonder, why?"

"To ask my sons, or my stepdaughter, or my father to help while I'm dying," insisted Mary, "that's a terrible burden to place on another human being. I couldn't stand the humiliation of them taking care of me as I faded into some useless and smelly dying person. And I certainly couldn't ask them to help me kill myself. Is that so unusual?"

Mary paused, looking out over the valley hanging below the forested path. "If we had more time," she said, "I'd take you through this beautiful chaparral forest, then back by the lake. I've walked up here a number of times since just after my chemotherapy, and thought, 'Well, maybe this is my last time up here.'" Mary walked on. "I've learned to stop thinking that way. I still have some responsibilities ahead. My mom taught me about dying, and it's my turn to pass it on to my kids."

As we walked up a narrow wooded path, Rosie now trotting comfortably close by, Mary talked about her mother. "Mom was nearly blind most of her adult life. And it didn't slow her down a bit. I never heard her say a word about her blindness." She hesitated, briefly lost in a memory. "Except one time," Mary began again. "When I was fourteen, she caught me reading a *True Romance* magazine. Boy, did she yell. 'You're wasting good eyes on that trash. You could be reading something useful.' My mom's whole family was pretty much that way. You take care of yourself, hold up your end of the stick. I was brought up not to lean on people for things I could do myself.''

"Like shooting yourself," I asked, "so as not to upset your family?''

Mary turned rapidly and stared at me. "I think the journalist part of me may like talking to you," she said. "But I'm not so sure how the rest of me is going to feel about it.''

Mary outlined dozens of reasons and methods she had formulated to protect her family from the hard times of her upcoming death. But she didn't speak of one thing—that most of them did not want the very protection she offered and had expressed their desire to participate more in taking care of her. "Maybe I just need to stay in control," Mary noted. "I just can't stand the thought of them seeing me in that condition.''

"So who are you making it easier for?" I ventured. "Easier for them, or better for you?''

Mary continued her brisk walk, but tears flowed down her face, and she did nothing to hide her sobs. Then she turned again to face me directly. "I don't know the answer to that," she said. "This conversation is getting to me. But I want to go on with it. I really haven't figured out the right way to do this death thing yet.''

She started walking back down the path toward home. "In all this confusion," Mary told me, "there is one thing I'm sure of: My family will have a lot more trouble dealing with their grief if they are feeling conflicted about what our relationship has been. So I have already made sure that, when the moment comes, we have said our good-byes and we are ready. I don't think I've got any relationships that are tied up in knots.''

Over the next two years, our initial verbal sparring smoothed out into a close friendship as we examined together the intricacies and significance of her planned suicide. After I met her stepdaughter Ann; Mary's father, Don; her cousin, and her writing friends, I couldn't help but agree that Mary might indeed have it right. There were no relationships still tied up in knots, and she could leave peacefully at the time of her choosing.

Yet it is still a mystery how, during those two years of my joining Mary, her family and friends, I never did manage to meet up with her son Paul Bowen and never heard from anyone the real story of the Bowen family. When I finally met Paul, at the very death scene that Mary had so dreaded, he was ready to have me physically removed from the hospital. And I still had not learned the secrets he held.

• • •

"I survived the bone-marrow transplant," said Mary, showing off her "diploma"—a blue-ribboned dog bone, framed and hanging on her office wall. "Unfortunately," she continued, "my cancer also survived." That May of 1991, it seemed clear to Mary that she would lose the battle with her cancer. She gathered her family about her to explain how she planned to die. Her brother Doug, a pathologist who lives on the East Coast, flew in for the meeting. Ann McGinley, Mary's stepdaughter from her eighteen-year second marriage, which had ended amicably, was there with her family. Steve Bowen, one of Mary's three sons from her first marriage, to Bob Bowen, drove over from the Sacramento Valley where the kids had been raised. His brother Paul, the youngest son, did not come up from Southern California for the meeting but kept in touch with the rest of the family, and with Mary, about what went on.

"It's not going to be easy to kill myself when the time comes," Mary told her father, Donald Cordray, an eighty-eight-year-old man who still shared camping and canoeing trips with his daughter. "I'm only certain of one thing," she added firmly. "I'll do the suicide by myself."

Her father showed no surprise. "You've always done everything by yourself," he stated calmly, still having a hard time realizing that at eighty-eight he was going to outlive his daughter and would greatly miss his favorite hiking companion. "Why should you change now?"

"I'm going to say good-bye to everyone," Mary continued. "But I want no formal, official good-byes around some bed when I'm really sick. We'll have all our good-byes over with, while I'm still well. And if I take a downturn, you all know what I'm going to do, and we'll already have had our parting. I'm not going to tell you when I'm going to do the suicide, so you'll just have to be prepared. You'll probably sense in general when the time is near, within a few weeks—but no one but me will know the specific day."

Only her brother Doug conveyed out loud his feelings about Mary's plan. "Mary," Doug said softly, "we hope it won't come to that."

She didn't halt for a moment. "Joining the Hemlock Society has been an important step for me," Mary told them. "What I'd really like to happen is to end my life when I'm very close to death, in that last week or so when it's really not even me anymore, and nothing but misery. That's the time I'd like to die." Mary sighed. "But that's not how it will happen," she declared. "Since my doctor is not allowed to help in my suicide, and I won't put anyone in this family through the ordeal of being there—that means I will have to die while I'm still strong enough to carry it out myself. And that will probably deprive me of a few months of good life."

It sounded like a well-thought-out plan, as would be expected from Mary Hall. And on that day no one in the family spoke out against it. Yet for all her wisdom, strength, stubbornness and planning, Mary could not foresee one crucial snag in her scheme. She had already been through many severe periods of illness from the cancer, each soon followed by a remission that allowed her to return to a comfortable life. How would Mary know which future recurrence of her cancer would be the *final* event, unless she waited to see if the illness progressed in severity, and possible agony, to where she was certain of death? "I don't mind the suffering," noted Mary, "if I know there's something more at the end of it." Chemotherapy, radiation, a bone-marrow transplant—at various times each kept death temporarily at bay. It added up to five years. Now, Mary's plan to kill herself "while still in midstride" would be tremendously difficult to carry out, not knowing how many months or even years she'd be giving up if yet another remission might come along.

Only time and experience would show Mary Hall if she really could end her life *before* she reached the state of suffering that would convince her she was truly, this time, at death's door. And if she did kill herself while still in midstride, could her family ever be reassured that the woman they so intensely loved had not mistakenly died too soon?

• • •

Mary's cancer started to grow again in November of 1992, after the temporary remission brought on by the bone-marrow transplant. This time, it showed up on her skin. First there was a scattering of small red blotches. Over months, it appeared as if she had hives, red welts all over her arms, neck, and chest—each one a cluster of millions of cells of breast cancer that now invaded her skin. This visible evidence became, for Mary, a tangible sign that she was finally approaching death.

At the same time, articles began appearing about a new wonder drug, Taxol, that was "curing" women who had ovarian cancer—a tumor with a well-deserved reputation for being aggressive and deadly. And studies were being started up to see if Taxol would work on breast cancer as well.

Strangely, Taxol had also become a new symbol for the environmental movement. The active chemical in Taxol could be found only in the bark of the Pacific yew tree. What better argument, claimed the environmentalists, for regulating the cutting of trees, to preserve the rain forests; who knew what other miracle drugs would be lost if we continued to lose entire species of plants? But for Mary Hall, the fact that Taxol could only be made from the rare yew tree simply added to her frustration. She considered the scarcity of the Pacific yew to be a personal insult.

"Knowing about Taxol," lamented Mary, "makes me feel even more vulnerable. They're teasing me. I know they're searching for a way to make more of the drug synthetically—but it'll be too late for me." Mary held out her arms, covered with red blotches of the cancer. "Taxol is a glimmer of hope on the horizon," she said. "It makes it even more difficult to deal with the finality of my death. I had my emotions all organized, and then Taxol comes along and I find myself scheming to try to get some, instead of getting ready to die."

The tumors on her arms, neck and chest enlarged slowly over the following months. For Mary, the red marks were a constant visual reminder that the cancer would eventually consume her. She began wearing long-sleeved, turtleneck sweaters, no matter how hot the weather, to avoid the sight of her own skin. "I'm the original illustrated woman," she said, "but who needs to look at it?" While various treatments seemed to slow the growth of the red welts, none stopped their inevitable spread.

By December of 1992, the skin tumors were large, increasingly swollen, and painful—as clear a sign as there could be that her cancer was advancing more rapidly. Mary talked with me about whether this might be the time, while still in midstride, to take her life.

Fortunately, she waited.

"If you want to be sure about things," Mary had said after

she'd recovered my lost dog, "go after them yourself." Although there was barely enough Taxol in existence to supply a few research programs, and thousands of women with cancer who wanted to try the drug, Mary contacted every medical center working with the medication. "I've started yapping and insisting on getting Taxol," she declared. "It's kind of psychotic. I'm fighting to get into some Taxol program, and at the same time I'm trying to figure out a way to kill myself." Mary was told repeatedly that she could not qualify for an experimental Taxol program, since she'd already had so many powerful cancer treatments that had weakened her body, and because her cancer was so far advanced. Yet she continued to contact one program after another.

Ironically, the very visibility of her skin cancers, a visual presence she had come to despise, became her saving grace. Physicians running an experiment with Taxol in San Diego, California, were looking for a few patients with breast cancer in whom they could easily observe the response, or lack of it, to the medication. When they heard about Mary's skin tumors, they saw a rare opportunity to watch and measure the effects of the drug. On January 6, 1993, Mary flew to San Diego and received her first intravenous infusion of Taxol, a chemical so caustic it had to be stored in glass containers and delivered to her body through specially constructed IV tubing. After her first dose of Taxol she became violently ill. But over the next few weeks, Mary literally watched her skin cancer disappear. The red blotches became more pale, less painful, as the cancer cells died. Within a month, she held her arms in front of her in astonishment; Mary had to search carefully to find any signs of the tumors.

"I have been practical and realistic about this cancer stuff," Mary declared. "But I'm becoming increasingly optimistic. It's hard not to be. I'm not sure Taxol is going to cure me, but I

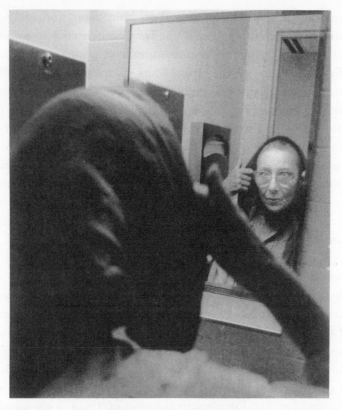

Mary Hall in the hospital during her
course of Taxol treatments.

think it's going to send me into a good, strong, long remission.''
With that, Mary Hall decided to make some significant changes
in her life.

• • •

''I don't like to impose on people,'' said Mary when she
considered, at age sixty, moving to a rest home, where the
average age of her neighbors was seventy-three, and the decor,
as she described it, consisted of ''visual Muzak.''

When the cancer erupted on her skin, Mary made an

offhand comment to her doctor about the home. "He told me, 'Why don't you move now?' " said Mary. "This did not cheer me up."

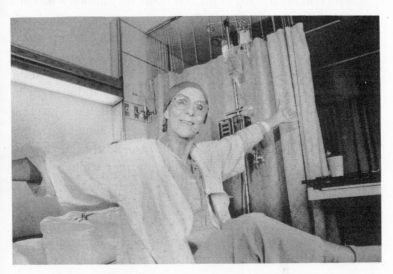

Mary celebrates the success of her Taxol treatments.

Mary moved into the enclosed rest home known as "the lodge," a large building that contained a number of apartments intended for the elderly and infirm to live out their last days, with ready access to a dining hall serving prepared meals, medical supervision, and, in every room, emergency buttons to push when help was needed.

She immediately hated it. "This place is an institution," she complained. "I resent the management's desire to have everyone coalesce and be convivial, I don't like having to eat my supper by six o'clock, and I feel a rather sophomoric urge to rebel against the whole place." Soon after Mary moved in, the ornate fountain at the entrance to the lodge began to spout water in elaborate colors. Someone, it seemed, was putting food dye in the recirculating water, a different color each day.

"Tacky," I said when I first noticed it. "Yes, very," replied Mary, keeping a straight face as she walked by the iridescent pink flowing water in the elegant fountain.

Mary had been living at the rest home for only a few months when she was accepted into the Taxol program. "After each dose of Taxol," recalled her close friend Arthur Jaseau, "she'd go back to her apartment and crawl from her bed to get to the bathroom to throw up. And then she'd clean it up. She never did push the button to get any help. She just didn't want to inflict her sickness on anyone else. In her mind, it was just that way. I find it very powerful in her, most commendable." After Mary's initial toxic reaction to the Taxol, the treatments continued with very few side effects, and her feeling of well-being soared. She stopped going to the rest-home dining room for meals and joined Arthur to head for the nearest Thai restaurant.

Mary had moved into the rest home thinking she'd die there. But when the Taxol beat back her cancer, her mood changed. She found the place tremendously depressing. At $1,835 a month, she also realized, "I think I'm going to live longer than my money will last after all." Mary moved out of the rest home and into a two-story condominium. "It's a matter of regaining control of my life," she said, standing in the hallway of her condo, teddy bear in hands, trying to figure out where to put all her family photos. And this time she did not hesitate to ask for help carrying her computer up the stairs to her new office so she could begin writing again.

When the Taxol made her skin cancers literally disappear, Mary Hall seemed like a child in a toy shop. She signed up for a mystery writers' conference that was scheduled a year in advance and sent in her check. She began work on a new book, this time nonfiction, about the history of women in California's Folsom prison. Mary spent days with a prison guard, exploring the still-functioning lockup. The guard told her how many killings and "knife stickings" there had been in each part of the prison, which had first opened in 1880. "It was a wonderful day," said Mary. "I really know how to party!"

During these times of Taxol-induced remission, Mary put her thoughts of suicide well into the background. "The cancer will be back someday," she acknowledged. "I'm not kidding myself about that. Taxol will not be some perfect happy ending to my story. But it's a wonderful extension of my life. I'll bring the suicide problem out to air again when the time comes. I'm sure I'll have plenty of warning."

· · ·

Tucked away in the back of Mary's mind were a number of rough sketches, all different, about her planned suicide. But for thirteen months after she'd started the Taxol, the idea of suicide floated in some limbo, waiting for the day when it might be needed.

"There is always that secret underlying hope that maybe the Taxol will get rid of this altogether," Mary told me at dinner in her house one evening. "There's some little hiding place where you keep that hope inside. I still know that dying is a problem to be solved, but I don't have to solve it now. I'm too busy living."

I got up from the table to get some ice and discovered that Mary's refrigerator freezer was packed with dozens of orange juice cartons filled with frozen water. "It's to keep the refrigerator cold in case an earthquake knocks out the electricity," she explained. "And with the added benefit of having water to use if that system goes out too."

"My God, Mary," I noted, "you're more prepared for an earthquake than you are for your own death." While Mary had thoroughly planned for the small possibility of a major earthquake, she had not even acknowledged the chance of an abrupt decline in her health from the cancer—a deterioration that might suddenly incapacitate her, eliminating the chance to finalize her plans for a "proper death." It made sense. In midstride, it was easy to prepare to survive an earthquake, impossible to plan how to die.

And yet in Mary's refrigerator, alongside the earthquake-readiness ice, were three other items of significance: two bottles of morphine and one of Darvon, the result of her incomplete research into possible methods of suicide, now on hold while the Taxol continued to work.

Even before the Taxol miracle came along, Mary had decided to reconsider the gun as her route to suicide. Her friend Arthur, who had trained in weaponry as a peace officer for the forest service, had appealed to her pragmatic side. "I know the damage a gun can do," Arthur told Mary during one of their dinner chats. "Whoever finds your body may be professionals, but even for them it's going to be one of the most gory and gruesome things, and a very difficult experience after racing on a 911 call in the hope of saving you. And they're not the ones who clean up the mess; someone in your family is going to have to arrange that, to clean the bathroom, replace the bathtub because it will get chipped and stained. And when your kids try to sell your condo they're going to have to explain over and over that their mom shot herself there. It's not good, Mary. You've got to think about all these things. You don't just finish it off by dying."

The conversation with Arthur convinced Mary at least to search for other possible methods she could use, alone, to guarantee her death. But it is more likely that Mary's eccentric sense of adventure, rather than Arthur's words, led her to explore other methods of suicide. Mary had learned about a retired CIA agent in favor of assisted suicide who had established contacts in Mexico to obtain lethal medications without prescriptions. She invited Mary to go down with her and smuggle the drugs back home.

Mary called me before she left for Mexico. "Does this mean

you've abandoned the gun idea?'' I asked. "Well, I thought I'd just have some backup plan," she responded, "and feel it out when the times comes. The lady who invited me is an ex-CIA agent, and the trip has this sort of rollicking aspect to it. Great, good, wild sport."

Mary Hall was not the first to head south on such an adventure. Soon after Derek Humphry had published his book of suicide stories with "hidden" drug recipes, *Let Me Die Before I Wake,* a group of Hemlock Society members from Tucson, Arizona, crossed the border and walked into Mexican pharmacies, overcoming the language barrier by carrying Humphry's book in with them and opening it to the pages with the names and dosages of the lethal drugs. It was not exactly a secret mission; CBS filmed it for *60 Minutes.* And possibly Mary and her ex-CIA friend, before leaving for Mexico themselves, missed a page in Humphry's next book, *Final Exit,* in the chapter titled "How Do You Get the Magic Pills?" "It has become more difficult," wrote Humphry, "to purchase suitable drugs in Mexico and Switzerland without a prescription. Perhaps Hemlock is the victim of it own members' news service; authorities over the border have become nervous."

Yet it was not the jumpiness of the authorities that was to make a farce out of Mary's trip to Mexico; as she would later admit, that was the fault of her own poor research.

Mary and her ex-CIA friend flew to Guadalajara, then walked into a pharmacy to ask for a bunch of harmless antibiotics; but added to their innocent list was an order for a lethal amount of the painkiller Darvon. The pharmacist filled the entire order, and after a few days of "boring tourism" they flew back home, Darvon in hand. The only problem, Mary discovered after arriving back in the States, was that Darvon, while highly toxic, was not certain to kill her. And an overdose of Darvon is also notorious for causing prolonged seizures, not a good way to die.

Yet the purchase of the Darvon did lead Mary, by an unplanned route, to finally secure Hemlock's coveted Seconal capsules—the Rolls-Royce of death pills. "I had never told my doctor about my specific plans for suicide," she declared, "until I got back from Mexico. I didn't want to put him under any pressure to help me, which he might have felt had I told him about the gun. And I didn't think it would work to lie to him—we knew each other too well. But when I returned from Mexico, now that I'd found my own means of doing it properly, I proudly told him about my Darvon cache." Mary's doctor stared at her in disbelief. He reminded her that about a year before, when she was having severe pain in her back from the tumor that had invaded her spine, he had given her a prescription for liquid morphine. "Mary," he said calmly, "the morphine is much more powerful and lethal than Darvon. And you've had it all this time." Mary flushed red with embarrassment. Sitting in the refrigerator at the home of this journalist and mystery writer, for well over a year, was just the type of medication she had flown all the way to Mexico to smuggle back into the country. But the biggest surprise was yet to come. "Mary," said her doctor, "you just needed to ask. When the time arrives, I will give you a prescription for Seconal."

After three years of planning, Mary had obtained a gun, two bottles of morphine, a large supply of Darvon, and the promise of a lethal dose of Seconal. She then fought her way into the Taxol program and promptly forgot about them all. "It's such a waste of time to work out the details now, and to talk to my family about it," said Mary. "I am still totally determined to take my life and don't need to decide now about timing, or pills or gun. I know from experience that I often formulate elaborate plans, and then when the time comes I do something entirely different."

• • •

In February of 1994, thirteen months after Mary started the Taxol treatments, she again noted faint red marks on her skin. Some tumor cells had become resistant to the Taxol. Within weeks, they were growing with a vengeance. "I've discussed this with my doctor," said Mary, "and he doesn't think anything terrible's going to happen right away. He's the perpetual optimist. But he did offer to write the prescription for Seconal. Tactless doctor. I took him up on it."

Mary started on yet another round of intensive chemotherapy to try to slow the cancer. The side effects were terrible. A month later she called me to announce, "This is the first day in ten that I haven't been at the hospital for a blood test, a doctor's appointment, a transfusion. I'm exhausted. Every time I get a dose of chemotherapy, I give up three weeks of my life because of the side effects. Today, I'm finally back to the strength where I can walk a bit. A little hike in the woods, slightly uphill. I'm getting back into it."

Along with her occasional "test hike," Mary began another pursuit. The drug RU-486, used in France for abortions and not yet available for ending early pregnancies in the United States, was being used by some U.S. researchers to treat breast cancer. The same hormonal effect of RU-486 that brings on abortion, they reasoned, might destroy breast-cancer cells. Mary, unsurprisingly, began contacting medical centers that were using RU-486. And she personally delivered the paperwork to her doctor so he could try to get her into a research program with the new drug.

I was about to leave the country for a month in Central America. The day before leaving, I drove up to have dinner with Mary. She had just arrived from a doctor's appointment and was holding on to her father's arm for support as she walked

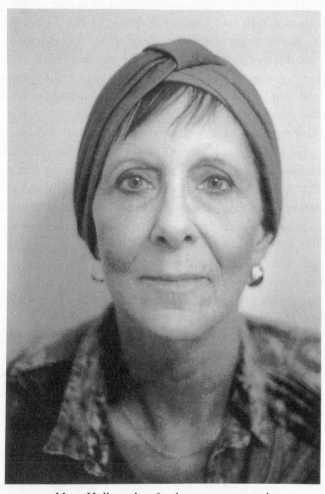

Mary Hall, weeks after her cancer recurred.

into her apartment. "Why don't you ask Dad what's going on," she said with no other greeting, slumping into a large, soft chair in the living room. "I haven't the strength to tell you about it."

The cancer had again invaded Mary's bones, this time damaging them so severely that calcium was leaking into her blood. Mary's calcium level was dangerously elevated. Any higher and she would become severely sedated, weak and confused. Fortunately, there were medicines to lower the blood calcium, and she had just started taking them. If the medications worked, her weakness would improve. If not, she would soon die.

Mary's father related the medical details to me while she rested. Then he left for a while, planning to return a few hours later and spend the night. Mary's physician, worried about her weakness from the elevated calcium, had insisted that she not be left alone.

"I need to bug my doctor about getting me into the RU-486 program," said Mary, her speech slurred, as if drunk, by her high calcium level. "Waiting even a few days can make a difference now," she declared. "I am hoping and praying that I can get into that program."

Weeks before, Mary's doctor had told her there was no chance at all, given the extent of her cancer, that any experimental program with RU-486 would take her in. He reiterated that opinion when she left his office that evening. But Mary had heard the same story more than a year ago, with Taxol, and had fought her way into the program. "I have to get to the point where I'm strong enough to walk again," she said, barely able to raise herself out of the living room chair to move to the kitchen table. "They won't take you into an RU-486 program if you are bedridden."

The next morning, I flew to Guatemala City, took a cab to Antigua, then called Mary at home to see how she was. There was no answer. I tried her father, no answer, and her stepdaughter Ann, only an answering machine. Then I tried the operator at the hospital near her house and asked for Mary Hall. "Four West," replied the operator, and she put me through.

"I think I'm OK," said Mary, "but I'm not too sure. Still fuzzy brained, hard to find some words. I'm in the hospital so they can treat the high calcium. But what really scares me is that being in the hospital may knock out any chance for the RU-486 program. They don't want anybody that's at the end of their rope." Mary sounded short of breath, and her speech was even more slurred than the last time we had talked. "I'm going to hang in here," she told me before hanging up, "and get strong enough to get into the RU program."

I called Mary again the next morning. The phone rang eight times, then a nurse answered, saying she'd have to hold the phone to Mary's ear for her to talk. "They have me strapped down," Mary explained. "I got out of the bed without asking for help last night, and I fell and hit my head. Now they have me strapped in so I won't do it again." There was a long pause while Mary tried to speak through her tears. "I'm tied to the bed rails," she finally managed to say. "Can you come back?"

"I'll be there tonight," I told Mary. "But listen carefully. Tell the nurses, tell them clearly, that you know you can fall, and that you will not leave that bed without help. Tell them, convince them that you have to be untied."

"OK," Mary said faintly, "I'll try my best."

I was shaking when I hung up the phone. I understood the real fears of the nurses and doctors, that Mary might fall if she tried to get up without assistance. By strapping her in the bed, they could prevent her from slipping and breaking her hip, or worse. But by tying Mary down to spare her body an injury, they most assuredly had killed her spirit. The night before, Mary had been fighting to get the strength to walk out of the hospital and into an RU-486 program. When they tied her down, she thought instead about suicide. "It's not death I'm afraid of," she'd said many times. "It's the process of getting there." Tied down, Mary faced her worst fears about dying. And she gave up.

When I arrived at the Los Angeles airport at 5:00 P.M. to switch planes on my way back to San Francisco, I phoned Mary again. "It's been a terrible day," she said. "I convinced them I would call anytime I needed to get out of bed, so they untied me. Now I've been calling for twenty minutes for help to get to the bathroom, and no one has shown up yet. I'll wait. I'll wait forever and shit in this bed before I'll let them tie me up again." Mary paused to catch her breath. "My family is here," she said, "and I've told them you're coming."

• • •

When I got off the elevator on the fourth floor of the hospital and walked to the cancer ward, Paul Bowen was waiting for me in front of the door to Mary's room. When he'd heard how sick his mother was, Paul had immediately flown up from Southern California. A slight man with a neatly trimmed beard, wearing jeans and a polo shirt, the thirty-four-year-old computer engineer looked worried but greeted me with a firm and friendly handshake. We chatted briefly, introducing ourselves. Although Paul talked in a soft and decidedly calm voice, I couldn't help but notice how rigidly he stood, and that his hands, hanging by his hips, were clenched into tight fists. And though his tone was gentle, Paul stood directly in front of the door to Mary's room, blocking the way. "I think I'll go in to see your mom now," I said.

Paul stayed in front of the door. "Let me tell you one thing before you go in," he said quietly. "I am completely, under any circumstances, against suicide. And I know why you're here."

Paul stared at the floor for a moment, then moved from the doorway.

Mary looked like she had aged ten years in the two days since I had last seen her. She was propped up in the hospital bed, thin oxygen tubing encircling her face. An intravenous line was attached to her arm. She was not tied to the bed rails, but they were carefully raised around her, and padded in case she might have a seizure. Her face was the color of chalk, and although lying still, she was breathing rapidly.

I closed the curtains around the bed, lowered one bed rail, and sat down on the edge of Mary's mattress, holding her hand. "We've got some business to take care of," she said without a pause.

Neither of us knew, as we began to talk about her plans for suicide, that Paul had silently come into the room and hidden himself behind the curtains, listening.

"I am not a violent man," Paul told me months later, "but I was ready to open that curtain and physically remove you from the hospital, or possibly put you in the hospital yourself, if I heard you tell my mother, as I expected you would, 'We've planned this for a while, Mary. Now the time has come.'"

"I guess it's time to decide," Mary told me.

"Mary," I responded slowly, "your doctor has told you what it will be like to die from a high calcium level. You will become more and more sedated, then unconscious, and then die. You're one of the fortunate ones. You're not in severe pain now, and it looks like you will have a comfortable death. Why do you still want to do the suicide?"

"Because I said I would," she replied.

"Mary!"

"I will do anything to further the Hemlock cause, because I have believed in it."

"Mary," I said, "your death is not some political act. The worst way to show that suicide at the end of life can be a rational choice is to do something as irrational as killing yourself simply because you planned to do it. You're not here to score political points, Mary, you're trying to find the best way to die."

"Oh," said Mary, fading out from the effort of even this

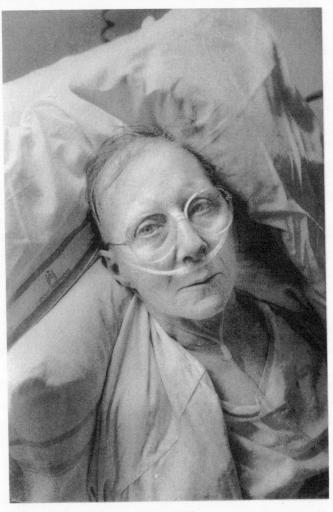

Mary Hall

brief discussion. Then she opened her eyes. "I guess I have some new things to think about. I had no idea that when the time came, things would move so fast. I need more time to think."

"You've got more time, Mary. There's no need to make any decisions. Your body is making the decisions for you."

Mary drifted off to sleep. I sat for a while, saddened by how rapidly Mary had become so ill. I heard the door swing open, and then close, and thought a nurse had come in to attend to the patient in the next bed. But it was Paul, quietly leaving the room.

• • •

"When my parents divorced," said Steve Bowen, the oldest of the three sons of Mary Bowen Hall, "it was like World War II, and take no prisoners." Steve paused, standing in the hallway with the rest of the family outside of the room where his mother was dying. "No," he thought, "they did take prisoners—the three sons."

"I guess I took the hardest fall when my parents divorced," observed Paul in a later conversation. "I was only eight, the youngest. And while my two older brothers chose to live with my dad, it was decided I'd be the one Mom would raise. I was miserable. Everything was going horrible at school, and at home. I was one unhappy guy. Mom finally agreed that I could go live with my dad and brothers. So my father came out in an old 1949 Ford pickup and loaded up my possessions. Before we went back to his house, he sent me in to see my mom and say good-bye. I didn't realize that would be the last time I would see my mother until I was seventeen."

Mary's dad remembers the divorce and loss of her children to their father, Bob Bowen, as the most agonizing time in Mary's life. "Before she lost her boys," said her father, Don, "she was softer, more lovable. Then she became a different character, and not for the better. She didn't laugh or play as much, became more impatient. It was very traumatic to Mary to be deprived of her children. And we were deprived of our grandchildren. We didn't see them for ten years.''

Mary's father attributes her loss of contact with her children to the difficulties posed by ''that miserable Bob Bowen.'' Paul, who remains close to Bob Bowen, acknowledged that his father may have been one part of the problem that blocked his mother from seeing her boys. ''My dad can be hard to deal with,'' he said. ''I can remember cowering in front of him at times.'' But no matter what the reasons for his parents' battles, to Paul, Mary's nine-year absence was an act of desertion. And it had left in him a deep and long-lasting emptiness. ''All I know,'' said Paul, ''is that for nine years I heard from Mom only when she'd send a birthday card. She averaged every three years or so. Not a letter, just a card.''

When Paul turned seventeen, he called Mary. ''She nearly dropped the phone when she heard my voice,'' he related. They agreed to meet for a walk in a nearby state park. When Paul arrived, Mary greeted him with a tight, long, and tearful embrace. Then Paul set the rules. ''We will never talk about what happened,'' he told Mary. ''Our relationship starts again at this day. I will not walk across the minefield of our past with you.''

From their reunion when Paul was seventeen, until just before his mother's death when he was thirty-four, Paul and Mary held fast to the rule of not treading through that minefield. In spite of many ''final hikes'' when Mary repeatedly told Paul, ''Let's make sure we don't have any loose ends in our relationship before I die,'' Paul did not speak of the times when they'd been apart. ''I wanted to remember my mother only as the woman I knew after we'd become close again, as adults,'' he said later. ''I couldn't deal with the rest of it. But I was left with a tremendous amount of unresolved pain.''

• • •

On the night of my arrival at the hospital to see Mary, her stepdaughter Ann invited the whole family to her house for dinner and some rest. Paul remained with Mary. "We should never leave her alone now," he said firmly.

While Paul stayed behind, the rest of the family moved to Ann's house. We all gathered around bowls of soup on the kitchen table.

"I guess the time has finally come," Ann commented to Mary's son Steve, "for Mary to decide about her suicide."

"I understand that she may want to do that," replied Steve, who describes himself as an evangelical Christian. "But my own feeling is that I believe in the hereafter. And my experience with suffering in this life is that quite often it's a tool to make a person grow. In the next few days, I think Mom may realize that. It would be an awful thing if she decided on the suicide just because she'd said she would. She's said it to so many people, I think she's feeling committed to carrying it out."

"Today," noted Ann, "I reminded Mary of my non-wedding to Michael. The family was there, the cake had come, I had my wedding dress laid out. Then a friend arrived, and we talked about how hesitant I was feeling. She said, 'Well, why don't you call it off?' It was just the permission I had needed to hear. I canceled the wedding at the last minute. And it was the best decision of my life."

Ann's husband, Tom, laughed. "And mine too," he said.

"I think the whole family needs to make it clear to Mary," said Ann, "that she's under no obligation to anyone to carry through with her plan."

"We have to be sure she knows that it's a dignified decision to decide *not* to kill herself," said Laura Bowen, Steve's wife. "But personally, I don't think she's going to buy it."

"My mom has lived for her books," said Steve, "and now

she's locked onto this crusade, and here's Lonny writing a book about her death. Books are everything in her life, and there's an audience out there. She has lived for that audience, and now she may decide to die based on what she thinks is the best ending for that audience."

"Frankly," said Ann's husband, Tom, "I don't think it makes a hill of beans difference whether she does the suicide now, or dies naturally. We're talking about just a few days, and they won't be very good days at that."

"I think the way she leaves us does make a difference," replied Steve, "in the way we'll remember her. It will be quite defining, really." Steve looked down at his hands, folded in front of him on the kitchen table. "Especially," he said softly, "for Paul and me."

The family agreed that the next morning each would emphasize to Mary that no prior commitment or philosophy should make her do the suicide. Her decision, they said, should be based on present reality, not past commitment.

"If she just sits tight," Ann thought out loud, "death will come peacefully to Mary soon enough."

• • •

Paul sat at his mother's side, watching her sleep. When she turned in bed, the pain of moving her cancer-ridden bones awakened her. Then she would notice Paul. "Each time she'd see me," he said, "Mom felt like she should talk. I realized I couldn't stay near her all night, or she'd never get any rest. I knew I'd have to get out what I wanted to say. But I just couldn't do it."

At midnight, Paul still sat silently, holding his mother's hand. "It took me a good fifteen minutes of crying before I could get the line out," he confessed. "I love you, Mom. You've been a good mother." Paul wiped his eyes, remembering his mother's reaction to his words. "Mom lifted herself up in the bed. I didn't think she had so much strength left to hug me that hard, that long.''

• • •

When I arrived early the next morning, Paul was sitting outside Mary's room; she was resting alone after the nurses finished bathing her in bed. The difference in Paul's mood was palpable when he greeted me. Although still filled with worry for his mother's comfort, his anguish, the taut desperation of the night before, seemed to have vanished.

"I'm sorry if I seemed harsh when we met last night," he told me. "I've had three friends who killed themselves; a man I'd known since our Cub Scout days hung himself. Horrible. Then I lost a girlfriend to a deliberate drug overdose. Another friend, just depression. And every time Mom talks about her suicide . . . I just don't know what to say. I don't think I could stand it."

A rustling noise came from Mary's room.

"Maybe you should go in," he said.

"I don't want to continue living like this," declared Mary when she saw me at her side. I anticipated another discussion about her suicide. "Maybe I could go home for a while," she announced, "do some more writing, finish up some business. When I'm done with that, I'll decide how to die."

"Mary," I said softly, "I don't think so."

"No," she replied. "I thought you'd say that." Mary turned her head to face me, grimaced from the pain of the movement, and managed a smile. "They can't just lower my calcium level, and then I walk home?"

"Your calcium level is back to normal now, Mary. But your bones are riddled with cancer, and the chemotherapy has made you severely anemic and susceptible to infections. Judging by how short of breath you are, your lungs are affected by the cancer as well."

"You're just filled with good news," replied Mary. Then she

looked straight at me. "Thank you," she said. "I need to decide, don't I."

Her panic hit before I could reply. She had rolled over to face me, grabbing the bed rail to pull herself up with one frail arm, suddenly crying out in pain from the twisting of her back. Paul came running in.

"I need to go," yelled Mary, shaking from the effort of balancing herself against the bed rail. "I need the bathroom, now!" and she began to crawl over the bed rail. Paul grabbed a portable commode and put it near the bed. He lowered the rail and lifted his mother in his arms, trying to carry her to the commode. Her pain was excruciating.

"Let me go!"—a deep cry of terror that seemed to come from someone other than Mary Hall and brought the nurses running. "I want help," shouted Mary. "No, let me out, get me out of this house!" Paul held Mary against his chest, her feet dragging along the floor. "I don't know what to do," he said to the nurses, his voice surprisingly calm.

"Get me off, get me out, let me go!"

Paul cradled his mother's head against his chest while she continued to scream into his body. He pleaded slowly, over and over, "Mom, it's Paul, please, Mom, it's OK, I'm holding you."

Briefly, the terror halted.

"Mom, do you know who I am?"

Mary looked up at his face, then said firmly, "You are my son Paul. Now for God's sake let me go. I want to be alone, and I will not be dragged to the bathroom to shit in front of my son."

Mary slumped in Paul's arms, and the foul smell of feces filled the room as she lost control and the loose stool ran out from under her diaper. She wept softly.

The nurse arrived with a sedative to inject into Mary's IV. "We can't control what happens if she panics like this," the nurse told Paul, who stood with legs braced apart, holding Mary's torso upright in his bear hug, his face against hers.

"Please," Mary cried out in anguish, her feet trying to find the floor. "I hurt, I hurt. It's running down my legs, for God's sake. Let me go."

The nurse began to inject the sedative. Paul's clear voice broke through his tears. "Do not do that," he addressed the nurse, pausing between each word. "Do not, please, do not give her anything that will keep her from thinking clearly. My mother said repeatedly that she wants to remain lucid. If that will knock her out, do not, please, do not inject it."

"We can't control her without this medication," repeated the nurse, nonetheless withdrawing the syringe that would have put Mary in a stupor for hours to overcome this moment of panic.

Paul carried Mary to the bathroom. "It's OK, Mom. It's me, Mom." Within a few moments the chant of her son calmed Mary. She relaxed in his arms as he placed her on the toilet, where he held her and cried and reassured his mother as the nurses removed the useless diaper and began to clean the now passive Mary Hall.

"I just didn't know what to do," Paul told me in the hallway as we waited for the nurses to finish their work and carry Mary back to bed.

"Paul," I said in awe, "you knew exactly what to do."

He wiped away his tears. "I never thought I could hold her and calm her like that," he said. "The time I had with Mom last night, and this morning, was very important to me." His tears flowed freely now. "I think it was important to Mom too."

• • •

"As I continue to deteriorate," Mary had told Ann when she first learned of her cancer, "it will be obscene to prop up what's left of me and have the family come take a look at it. So I've arranged to die before that."

Paul and I waited in the hall for the nurses to finish their

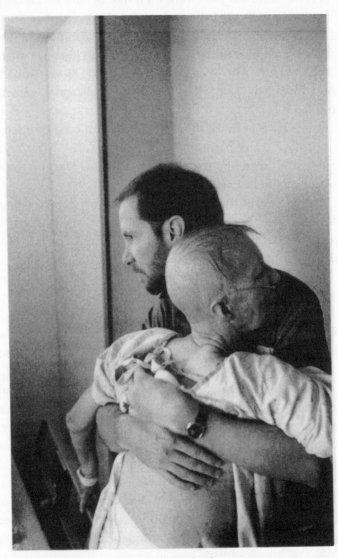

*"Mom, it's Paul, please,
Mom, it's OK, I'm holding you."*

work. Steve and Ann joined us, then one by one we filed in to visit with Mary. During the rest of the day twenty-two friends and family members came to see Mary and wish her good-bye. At times she slept, at others she awakened with pleasure to greet and chat briefly with cousins, friends, Paul, Steve, Ann, her second husband, Tom Hall, and writer colleagues who had heard she was ill.

"I will have none of those dreaded emotional farewells at the bedside," Mary had said three years before. "Where's my dad? I haven't seen him yet today," proclaimed Mary on the day the family gathered around her deathbed.

"I don't think the reality of what Mom's experiencing is what she predicted," observed Paul. "I had my turn to find some peace last night and this morning. I think the rest of the family is getting their chance today."

"She's gone downhill so suddenly," noted virtually every visitor as they left Mary's room. "I'm glad I came."

"I think Mom underestimated the amount of love and caring, the adulation, that was out there for her," asserted Paul. "I think she's realizing how much people really need to be with her today. I'm happy for her."

At various times in the day, I joined the group around Mary's bed. "I guess I should decide," Mary would say each time she saw me. My presence had become the last reminder of her planned suicide. "Mary, you don't have to decide anything," I responded automatically, and took to staying in the corners of the room, out of her field of vision.

At 5:00 P.M., Paul sat by his mother's side while she rested. She opened her eyes occasionally to see that he was there. Then Paul kissed his mother and left the hospital to return home. I walked with him to where a cab waited for the drive to the airport. "My wife is away at a conference," he said, "and my two-year-old, Julia, is at child care." He shook my hand good-bye, then moved to an embrace. "I don't like to leave Julia alone for so long."

• • •

By 6:00, the visits ended. Only Mary's closest family remained around her bed. Ann and Tom McGinley; Steve and his wife, Laura; Tom Hall; Don, her father; and her stepdaughter Rita. Exhausted by the day of farewells, Mary slept, briefly awakened by her painful movements. The family stood around the bed, talking quietly.

I left to spend some time alone in the waiting area of the cancer ward, thinking of my last two years with Mary. I was the only one who knew of the bottle of Seconal she'd hidden in the bedside drawer when she arrived at the hospital. Mary, I was certain, was moving slowly into a peaceful death. There'd be no need for the Seconal.

"Come quickly." Ann startled me. I followed her back to the room.

Mary was wide awake, sitting up in bed, eyes glaring. In her left hand, held aloft like a banner, she grasped the oxygen tubing that she had removed from around her face. Mary saw me but said nothing.

"Mom has told us she's ready to die," explained Ann.

"You've all had your farewells," declared Mary. "What are we going to do for the next days while I wither away, say good-bye over and over again?"

Ann turned to me. "Will you talk with her?"

I moved to sit at Mary's side. The family remained gathered at the foot of her bed.

Mary stared defiantly. "Why are you so scared for me to do this?" she addressed me.

"Mary," I replied, "from everything we can see now, you will die a comfortable death within the next few days—"

"How can you say I'll die comfortably," she broke in, "when I'm so disgustingly uncomfortable now?"

"Maybe your doctor can help with that," I offered. "What's making you so uncomfortable?"

"Everything."

"Don't be so eloquent, Mary Bowen Hall," I replied, using the full name she used as an author. Her tension seemed to ease, and Mary lowered her left arm, though still holding in her hand the oxygen tubing she was refusing to wear.

"I am miserable," she said softly, her anger dissipating. "I don't mind the pain, although it's pretty bad moving around. It's just that I can't do anything."

"What about conversations with your family?"

"That's been fine, for a couple of days. We've said what we've had to say." Mary looked at the clan gathered by her bed. "If I could find any reason to go on with this, I would," she told them. "But there is nothing to be gained by anyone from these next few days of my misery."

Mary was becoming increasingly short of breath, her lips blue from lack of oxygen.

"Mary," I said, "please put your oxygen back on. There is no comfort in dying by suffocation. And we can't be sure you're thinking clearly when your brain is lacking oxygen."

"There is nothing good in this situation," she responded, becoming agitated again. "I am frustrated as hell, and I am ready to end this." She stared at me. "And I will not put on my oxygen."

"Mary, we, your family, me, you . . . we have to understand this. Slow down a bit. Put on your oxygen, and I will leave you alone with your family for a while. That's not asking so much. When I return, we'll talk about your suicide."

Mary put on the oxygen tubing. "Fine," she said. "But when you come back, I am going to do it. It is ridiculous and humiliating for me to lay here dying for days. There is no quality left to my life and nothing left that I need to do." She looked at Ann, then at her son Steve. "I am grateful for these last days," she said. "But I don't need any more."

Forty-five minutes later, I returned to Mary's room.

Steve Bowen was the first to speak. "We agree," he said simply.

"You mean you'll support her decision?"

"No," said Steve after a moment's thought. "Months ago, or yesterday, we would have supported her right to make this decision. But we wouldn't have agreed with it. Now, we agree. Tonight, seeing the way things are, I not only support my mother's decision, I understand why she is making it. We're tremendously sad, but we are ready."

I looked around the room. Everyone nodded in agreement. Only Mary's father was not there. The eighty-eight-year-old man, exhausted, had gone home. And Paul, who perhaps had the most at stake in this decision, was on an airplane en route to Santa Barbara.

Mary's family, one by one, went to her side for a kiss on the cheek, a brief embrace. Then they left the room.

Ann, in tears, was the last to leave. "Sister, mother, friend," she whispered as she held Mary tightly against her, "I love you."

• • •

"You stay," Mary told me. "We've got a job to do, and you signed up a long time ago. Besides"—she managed a soft smile—"I don't think Paul would want me to be alone."

Mary reached into the bedside drawer, took out the bottle of Seconal and poured the capsules into her hand. Without warning, the door to the room swung open. It was Tom, Ann's husband. He motioned for me to talk privately with him outside the room.

"What happens if one of the nurses comes in while she's

still holding a bunch of sleeping pills?" he asked. "It might take a while to get them all down."

"Then they will take away her pills," I replied, "and put her under strict observation."

Tom seemed upset. "I'll stay here," he declared, "and distract the nurses in conversation if they're about to enter the room."

"Thank you," I responded, and returned to Mary's side. She placed one Seconal capsule in her mouth at a time, sipping water with each pill. When she reached the last of the thirty capsules, she looked straight at me, nodded her head, then swallowed it down.

Mary lay back on the pillow, eyes open, waiting. An hour later, she was deeply unconscious. In a few more hours, she would stop breathing.

Ann entered the room with her twelve-year-old son, Jeff, Mary's grandchild, and Yori, the ten-year-old daughter of Mary's stepdaughter Rita. "They were at my house," explained Ann, "and I told them Mary was unconscious and would possibly die soon. Both asked if they could see her one more time. It seemed important."

The two children stood at Mary's side, watching quietly. Then Jeff reached out and placed a book, *The Hitchhiker's Guide to the Galaxy,* under his grandmother's folded hands. "Bye, Grandma," he said. "Glad I got to see you again."

"Have a good time in heaven," added Yori, but it was only when they all reached the door that I heard the girl say quietly, "I love you, Grandma."

• • •

I drove over to Ann's house, where the family was gathered. "We're OK," Ann greeted me, with a tearful embrace. We all sat for a while, talking about Mary and the times we had spent with her.

As Ann walked me to the door, we spoke of our concerns for Paul. "He wasn't there when Mary decided on the suicide," she said. "I'm not sure how he's going to take it. Steve is calling him now to talk it over."

The next morning I phoned Paul to offer my condolences. We both felt it was too soon to discuss the details of how his mother had died, but easily talked about our shared sorrow. Paul had spoken at length with Steve about the events of Mary's final night. Yet I was still worried about how unsettled he might feel. Three months later I drove to Santa Barbara to spend a day with him, and to meet his wife and daughter.

Paul greeted me warmly as he led the way out to the sunny back patio of the modest but comfortable home he had bought and renovated in the coastal hills of Southern California, ten minutes from where he and his wife worked as computer engineers. When Julia, his rambunctious two-and-a-half-year-old daughter, came running out, I suddenly remembered that Mary had left for this favorite grandchild a music box, bequeathed to Mary when her own grandmother died.

Mary had told me the family's favorite fable. "When I was sick," she recounted, "Grandma would wind up this music box, and I would lay very still. When the music box ran down, I'd be asleep. And when I woke up, I'd be well again."

Mary's granddaughter toddled off to run through the playground Paul had built in the backyard. Her father watched carefully, then said to me abruptly, "I think I will regret for the rest of my life that I left the hospital that day."

I anticipated what he was feeling. "Paul," I offered, "I don't think there was anything you could have done to stop it."

"I know that," responded Paul, smiling at my misunderstanding. "I'm just so sorry that I missed my mother's finest hour."

"I'm not sure I'm following you."

"Mom's suicide," Paul continued, this time not flinching at

the very word, as he had when I'd seen him last, "gave her a good death." Paul hesitated. "Don't get me wrong. The night before, or even during the next day while I was still there, I would have done anything I could to have stopped her suicide. There was so much we still had to say, and she was making such good contact with people. I needed those last moments with her, and I would have been angry forever if she had taken them from me."

Paul's tears made it difficult for him to talk. We stopped for a while. "I'm not crying because of the way she died," he told me. "I'm crying because I miss her. I had wanted for so long to tell my mother what I finally said during that last night with her. 'You've been a good mother.' But until I knew clearly that this was my last chance . . . I just couldn't get the words out. There was so much I was still angry about. In a lot of ways she wasn't a good mother; but in so many ways she was."

Paul's wife joined us, sitting next to him in the sun on the patio, watching Julia play, and lightly touching Paul's hand as he continued. "The night before Mom died, when I stayed up with her, I believed her decision for suicide was wrong. She was lucid, not in severe pain. And she had an obligation—I really believe that—not to deprive us of those final moments. She had so much still to offer us. If she had killed herself that night, it would have been torture. But you see, we all learned something. It didn't matter how Mom died, by suicide or not; what mattered most was the timing. Not just for us, but for Mom as well."

"What changed in that brief time?" I asked.

"If Mom had killed herself the night before, it would have been a suicide," concluded Paul, "just like the horrible suicides of my friends. She was ending a life that still had meaning. She wasn't propped up half dead, she was giving a lot to her friends and family. The person, Mary Bowen Hall, was there, with reasons to be alive. I don't think anybody would have wanted to lose that time. But by the next night I truly believe the meaning

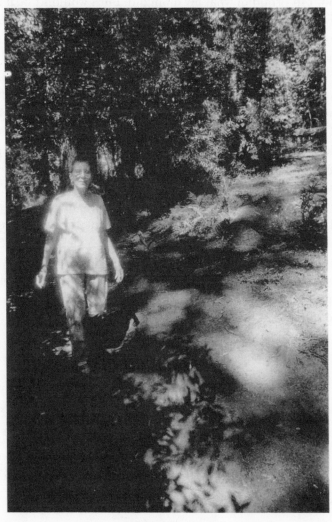

Mary Bowen Hall

was gone for her. By the time Mom took the pills, there were only hours left, at most one or two days. And there was no more to do. I'm proud of what my mom did. But I wouldn't be if she had ended her life just twenty-four hours sooner. The important question wasn't whether or not she did the suicide—it was the timing of it. We all needed that last day."

Then Paul looked at his wife and uttered the words that surprised us all. "The night before," said Paul, "I would have done anything to keep my mother from taking those pills. But had I still been at the hospital that next evening, and Mom looked me in the eye and said, 'Paul, I need your help, I've got to go and I can't do it myself . . .' I would have helped in my mother's suicide."

Paul hesitated, trying to understand fully what he had just said. "Mom wasn't the only one that went through changes when faced with the reality of this situation," he decided. "She wanted so much not to linger. And if the doctors wouldn't do it, I would have helped her die. But it would be the most painful thing for the rest of my life—what a horrible thing for a son to have to do."

Chapter Six

Hospice and Hemlock:
A Plan

———

[T]his question [of euthanasia] should be speedily discussed; so that in case any change should be thought possible and right, that change might occur in our lifetime.

—PHILOSOPHER LIONEL TOLLEMACHE, 1873

The 1990s is the decade when the issue of voluntary euthanasia for the terminally ill will be decided . . . In the name of compassion, let the debate not go on for too long.

—DEREK HUMPHRY, 1992

With widespread availability of good hospice care for the terminally ill, the question of euthanasia would become moot. People simply don't want euthanasia when they are physically comfortable and their emotional needs are addressed.

—DR. DAVID CUNDIFF,
hospice physician, in *Euthanasia Is Not the Answer*

Those who have witnessed difficult deaths of patients on hospice programs are not reassured by the glib assertion that we always know how to make death tolerable.

—DR. TIMOTHY QUILL,
hospice physician, in *Death and Dignity*

"When the nurses I work with at hospice tell each other they've got an impossibly difficult patient," said Clarissa Ramstead, the thirty-four-year-old hospice nurse who had been assigned to work with Pierre Nadeau, "we just do the Pierre imitation." Clarissa covered her face with her palms, then slowly lowered them so that only her brown eyes peeked out, peering back and forth over the tops of her fingers. "When I first walked into Pierre's room and told him I was the nurse from hospice," she explained, "he pulled the blankets over his head. Then his eyes appeared just over the edge of the covers; and I remember the first thing he said to me: 'Go away.'" Clarissa laughed. "It was a pretty awful beginning with the guy who turned out to be my most successful patient."

Pierre had just returned home to Gordon's house from the hospital, and he was sorry to still be alive. On the walls of his room hung framed portraits of dancers and other performers, beautiful bodies in wondrous positions of grace.

"Pierre was really angry that we hadn't killed him while he was in the hospital," recalled Gordon. "He'd had an IV attached, and he wanted us to take advantage of it and just inject all his morphine." But Gordon and Stephen had rejected this proposal. And Lynn demanded that Pierre wait it out for one more month, until Alexa arrived. Although Pierre agreed, he also let everyone know how miserable he was with the decision. To make matters worse, Gordon insisted on getting help to care for Pierre at home; he arranged for a hospice nurse to come to the house.

"Pierre," said Gordon, "don't blow this. If you tell her you've got a plan for suicide, she's either going to take your medicines away and turn you in, or she just won't come back."

Gordon knew almost nothing about hospice when he delivered that warning to Pierre. And he had no idea at all that he'd just stepped into the center of an intense war being waged by hospice organizations around the country against laws that might establish the right of a dying patient to have assistance in suicide.

"We are instructed," Clarissa told me in a conversation a year after Pierre died, "that if a hospice patient has a firm plan for suicide, we absolutely must intervene. This results at least in taking away medicines that he might use for an overdose, or hospitalizing the patient against his wishes and getting him psychiatric help; we ask the patient to either come in on his own, or we will send an ambulance crew to pick him up. Hospice believes that if you give people enough time and stop patients who are trying to take their lives, they will come to terms with their demons and be able to have a peaceful death. The transformation to peace and acceptance is part of the process of dying." Clarissa looked at the microphone that was recording her comments. "OK," she conceded, her tone lightening, "so much for official hospice policy. Now let's face reality. Not everybody can have the death that we read about in hospice textbooks."

Clarissa Ramstead, an ex–marine biologist turned nurse, with intensely specialized hospice training to care for the dying, hesitated before she continued. "Boy, will I get into trouble with hospice for saying this stuff," she thought out loud. "For some people, dying can be very different than this organization wants to project. I've seen some really horrible deaths. We are great at helping almost everybody along, both physically and emotionally," Clarissa sighed, "but we just can't fix everybody."

Then Clarissa backtracked. "Don't get me wrong. When I first met Pierre he was sitting in bed staring at the wall. I couldn't get him to say anything more than yes or no. That was in March. Before he died in July, I was blown away by how courageous a transformation he'd gone through. If I ever get to the point where Pierre was, I hope I can be as strong and do it with as much dignity as he did. Pierre was this fairy-tale hospice story; he showed it can really work.''

• • •

In 1957, Dr. Cicely Saunders entered the Our Lady ward at St. Joseph's Hospital in London and began her pioneering work on how to relieve the pain—both spiritual and physical—of patients dying from cancer. St. Joseph's was founded in 1905 by the Irish Sisters of Charity and the hospital had "come to represent a blend of spirituality and hard medicine." At St. Joseph's, Dr. Saunders, described as a "deeply committed Christian," had such remarkable success in easing the death throes of so many suffering patients that in 1967 she moved to the London suburb of Sydenham and founded St. Christopher's Hospice. Here she began an uphill battle for the acceptance of her new principles by which to treat people who are dying. Instead of aggressive attempts to keep patients alive as long as possible, no matter what their condition, Dr. Saunders thought that in every death there comes a time to withdraw the high-tech hospital care that sustained life, and then to mount an equally intense effort to make people as comfortable as possible as they moved toward their inevitable death.

It wasn't an easy battle for Saunders. Most physicians at the time felt that withdrawing life-prolonging treatments, such as deciding not to use antibiotics to treat a serious pneumonia in a patient dying from cancer, was the same as killing the patient. In essence, Dr. Saunders was arguing that patients should be allowed to decline all treatments, except those that would make them comfortable, and to move rapidly and with less suffering to their natural death.

To keep her critics at bay, and because of her own staunch religious and philosophical beliefs, Saunders always emphasized that she did no more than to allow the patient to die naturally— never anything to speed up the process. "Hospice neither hastens nor postpones death" became the slogan repeated time and again by those advocating the benefits of hospice care. "Hospice affirms dying as part of the normal process of living and focuses on maintaining the quality of remaining life."

Cicely Saunders and the hospice movement did more than simply plead that suffering patients should finally be allowed to die; the main strength of hospice came from its aggressive and meticulous attention to treatments that could make the process of dying as comfortable—even rich and rewarding—as was possible. Saunders initiated the concept that pain should be prevented, not just treated when it became intense. Rather than wait for a person to cry out in pain and then give them medication for it, hospice practitioners learned to anticipate the agony and administer adequate doses of narcotic pain relievers *before* distress became severe. And fears of narcotic addiction were thrown to the wind when research showed that dying patients did not abuse the drugs but used them to achieve comfort. Saunders also demonstrated that skilled adjustment of narcotic dosages would allow most patients to control their pain without the side effect of heavy sedation.

"People in hospices," wrote Sandol Stoddard in her book *The Hospice Movement: A Better Way of Caring for the Dying,* "are not attached to machines, nor are they manipulated by drips or tubes, or by the administration of drugs that cloud the mind without relieving pain. Instead, they are given comfort by methods sometimes rather sophisticated but often amazingly simple and obvious; and they are helped to live fully in an atmosphere of loving-kindness and grace until the time has come for them to die a natural death." Most significantly, hospice actively involved both patient and family in making decisions about what treatments should be used, or withheld. In the 1960s, asking patients about their own medical care was a radical concept. Physicians wanting to maintain their control resisted Saunders' methods at every turn.

Dr. Cecily Saunders was adamant, some might say obsessed, in proving that her ideas and methods could change the final months of life into a period of transformation rather than suffering. And she was remarkably successful in her campaign. But descriptions of death under the care of her hospice team soon began to take on mythic proportions. Sandol Stoddard, a leading advocate of the international hospice movement, described the scene at St. Christopher's Hospice: "Azaleas, ferns, chrysanthemums, cyclamens, African violets. Two single rooms at the end of each hall, four beds in each large and airy bay, each with its own curtains that can be drawn shut, and each with its own furnishings around it . . . Colored quilts, knitted coverlets, and plenty of down pillows on each bed. Fresh white linens, worn and soft. Letters, newspapers, cigarettes, lamps, baskets of fruit. A bottle of port and two glasses. A family of five walking by with a small, gray dog padding agreeably along behind them on a leash. Beside the bed of an elderly woman in pink, a small girl is curled up in an armchair, sucking her thumb and reading a comic book."

Cecily Saunders and her supporters may have gone overboard in describing the wonders of hospice care. But if her public relations were overstated, her methods of treating the dying were sound, and they spread worldwide. By 1993, in the United States alone, 250,000 dying patients were cared for in hospices that followed the fundamental rules and principles of the now Dame Cecily Saunders.

But both Dr. Saunders and other hospice advocates and practitioners had become so involved in their long and crucial battle for acceptance that it was hard, if not impossible, to admit that even hospice had its failures. If hospice would only be allowed to do its work, they argued, patients' desires and requests for assisted suicide or euthanasia would simply disappear. The philosophy that "Each patient is unique and comes first in considerations of how to meet her or his individual needs" seemed to evaporate when some rare, severely ill individuals rejected prolonged life even under the best of hospice care—and asked for help to bring on their deaths. In 1991, the National Hospice Organization in the United States issued a position paper declaring without equivocation that it "rejects the practice of voluntary euthanasia and assisted suicide in the care of the terminally ill." Yet in the same statement, the National Hospice Organization reaffirmed the basic principles of hospice, which has "championed the ideals of relief of suffering, freedom of choice, and death with dignity." The organization made no mention of what should be done with the few patients for whom even hospice could offer little relief from intense suffering. In fact, some of the staunchest advocates of hospice care will not even admit that such patients exist.

• • •

When Renee Sahm's cancer had spread to her neck and weakness and dehydration brought on her collapse at home, she was admitted to the hospital's hospice unit. In the family room of the hospice there were large sofas, a refrigerator in which family and patients kept favorite foods, a small cooking area, a television, board games like Monopoly, chess, and checkers. The decorator, it seemed, had in mind the typical living room of a middle-class American home. Although there was no "bottle of port and two glasses," and the chrysanthemums and cyclamens were lacking, it was a surprisingly pleasant place, separated from the large main hospital building by a garden path and a small stone bridge over a quiet running creek. After I visited briefly with Renee, I rested in the family room for a moment, fixing a cup of tea. Down the hall, at my insistence, the nurses were untying Renee from the bars of her bed.

Confused and disoriented from her severe dehydration, Renee had spent the night screaming and trying to crawl over the bed rails to go home. To protect her from injury, she'd been sedated and tied down. By the next morning, Renee was less confused, yet by 10:00 A.M. she was still tied to the bed. "These were just a gentle reminder that you shouldn't leave the hospice without saying good-bye," the nurse explained to Renee as she took off the restraints that had become the worst part of her night of terror. Renee was then able to walk about the hospice ward, even sit in the garden in the sun. But there was only one thing on her mind. "I'll do anything to get out of this place," she told me. "I've heard about this part of the hospital, it's the place you never check out of."

Renee had it wrong. Hospices in the United States are intensely focused on trying to care for a patient at home. The hospital hospice unit where Renee was taken for brief intravenous treatment of her dehydration had been a last resort. The hospice team had every intention of getting her home as soon as they could arrange for Renee to have help there—regular visits from hospice nurses, aides, and social workers. The concept that patients should be able to die in the familiar surroundings of their own home was a major victory for hospice advocates in this country and is now well accepted by physicians who previously thought that all dying patients required hospital care.

Since Renee had no family (but fortunately adequate amounts of money), the hospice team helped her find a full-time attendant to stay with her at home. Hospice aides and nurses visited regularly, and their efforts were superb. They gently bathed Renee, instructed her attendant in schedules of medications, taught Renee the best way to eat and sip fluids to keep strong and avoid becoming dehydrated again, and how to adjust her medications to diminish the pain from the cancer spreading rapidly in her neck. Renee, as best she could, became content. "I really have just one major problem they still won't take care of," she told me. "The nurses keep calling me 'Sweetheart.' My God, I am forty-one years old, not one of their little eighty-year-old ladies!"

A week later Renee's hallucinations and panic set in. Scorpions crawled about her room; over and over, she shouted in fear during the same imagined plane crash. Renee tossed violently about in her bed while friends and her attendant provided a twenty-four-hour watch—knowing that the only alternative to the hallucinations would be heavy pharmacologic sedation. But while Renee had still been coherent, she'd spoken adamantly against this very sedation. Her friends agreed: Since she was slipping in and out of periods of coherence, heavy sedation might deprive Renee of important final lucid moments. But we all acknowledged it might eventually become too difficult to take care of Renee at home. The backup plan offered by the home hospice team was to take her again to the hospital's hospice unit. The treatment for her delirium there: physical and pharmacologic restraints.

"Patients who opt for euthanasia may miss the opportunity to transcend their suffering and find meaning in their lives for themselves and their survivors," states the National Hospice Organization's position paper against euthanasia. When Renee's friend Celia arrived, her very presence put a temporary halt to Renee's hallucinations, and the pair had a remarkable final day together. The hospice philosophy seemed clearly correct. Had Renee followed through on her planned suicide before Celia's visit, the two friends would have missed that most important time. But the same would have been true had Renee been sedated to unconsciousness to avoid the agony of her intermittent hallucinations. Her suffering through the hallucinations had been, by Renee's own account, made worthwhile by her chance to say good-bye to Celia.

Yet in the end, Renee made her own decision that she needed no further "opportunities to transcend suffering and find meaning" in her life, at the expense of the repeated hallucinations, or chemical sedation and possible physical restraints until her natural death would finally arrive. "Hospice neither hastens nor postpones death" was the choice of hospice. A hastened death was the choice of their patient, Renee Sahm.

All discussions about the possibility of Renee's suicide had to be hidden from the hospice team that was caring for her. "If they don't approve of suicide," said Renee, "they don't have to kill themselves. But I have one freedom left, and I gain nothing by this waiting around to die." The hospice nurses, those who might best have explained to Renee that there were better choices than suicide, had by their own rules and regulations been cut out of the crucial discussions while Renee considered killing herself. Hospice's firm policy to intervene against all attempts at suicide forced Renee not to speak to them of her plans, and thus not to receive their crucial input into her decision. By so vehemently opposing any individual's choice for suicide, hospice eliminated their chance to tell Renee, when she most needed it, of the better alternatives they might offer.

•   •   •

Clarissa carefully rolled Pierre over in his bed, searching his skin for early signs of pressure sores that she might prevent from forming, rather than having to treat them once they appeared. Hospice training taught Clarissa to anticipate the painful problems that can develop in bedridden patients. Noting how swollen Pierre's legs had become, Clarissa discussed the possibility of chemotherapy to temporarily reduce the size of the lymph nodes that kept the fluid from draining from his legs. "Chemotherapy is no cure for your disease," she said, "so it seems an aggressive thing to do. But you'll be more comfortable if we can decrease the swelling in your legs." Months after Pierre first told Clarissa to "go away," he came to completely accept the physical and emotional comfort, and the compassion and experience, of this stranger. The two developed a relationship that more resembled the love and trust of brother and sister than it did nurse and patient. But as with many brothers and sisters, there was a dark family secret they could not even discuss.

"It's so tricky," said Clarissa. "Of course I knew Pierre had plans for suicide. But if I asked him to talk about them, and he had, then I would have to do something about it. And that would have ruined my relationship with him, his trust in me. I mean, I can understand why my clients might see suicide as an option; but the system doesn't allow us to let them have that option—that is, if they inform us of it."

"Clarissa sat down with me," recalled Gordon, "and just said flat out, 'If you know something about Pierre's plans for suicide, please don't tell me. I know he's got *Final Exit*—it's the book of the day for my patients. But I don't want to hear any details.' "

"There are over half-a-million people out there reading *Final Exit*," commented Dr. Gary Johanson, a physician with fourteen years of experience with hospice who recently left to work in an independent community cancer clinic. "Those half-million people know that hospice can provide them with good care, but they want to keep the option open for suicide if things don't work out. And because of hospice's strong stand against that possibility, those patients will not go to hospice now. So they will lose the benefits of hospice's expert care." Dr. Johanson paused in frustration. "That's my worst fear. Hospice is a fantastic alternative and eliminates the need for suicide nearly all the time. But it's not right for everybody, and it doesn't work for everybody.

Hospice tells patients they can alleviate their suffering, so there's no need to consider the possibility of suicide. Well, the definition of suffering, of course, is up to the individual patient. And if patients run away from hospice because they want to keep open the possible option of suicide, then more people will be denied the benefits of hospice care—and more patients will need the alternative of suicide. It's like we're cutting off our nose to spite our face."

Dr. Johanson, who sits on the board of the Academy of Hospice Physicians, is one of a number of doctors with extensive hospice experience who have begun to break away from the long-standing hospice position against physician-assisted suicide. The debate among the leadership of hospice centers on one controversial issue: Is hospice really as good as it says in preventing the enormous suffering that can at times accompany death?

"We have the knowledge and the means to assure that no terminally ill person need beg for death to end his or her suffering," says Dr. David Cundiff, a hospice physician and author of the book *Euthanasia Is Not the Answer.* "Those patients who have asked me for assisted suicide or euthanasia," claims Cundiff, "have changed their minds once I took care of their symptoms. By all accounts, requests for assisted suicide are cries for help, not requests for death." Dr. Cundiff attributes the recent wave of public interest in assisted suicide not to the suffering inherent in death, but to physicians' uniform lack of knowledge in how to alleviate that suffering. Cundiff's point is crucial: Improved care of pain for those who are terminally ill is desperately needed.

"With the single exception of hospice care," writes Dr. Christine Cassel, Chief of Internal Medicine at the University of Chicago School of Medicine, "the medical profession is woefully ignorant of and unable to conduct compassionate comfort care . . ." And there is hard data to back up Cassel's claim. A

1993 survey showed that "doctors and nurses . . . say they often fail to provide adequate pain relief for dying patients in hospitals, despite that patient's expressed wishes to be spared severe pain." Another study published that same year in the *American Journal of Public Health* found that 81 percent of hospital nurses agreed that "the most common form of narcotic abuse in caring for dying patients is undertreatment of pain." Even specialists in cancer care receive minimal training in pain control. In a review of five thousand pages from textbooks on the care of cancer patients, only twenty pages referred to the management of pain. And on the lengthy board examination taken by cancer doctors to receive specialty certification—an exam filled with questions about the appropriate use of chemotherapy, surgery, radiation—there are no questions at all that test the cancer doctors' knowledge of how to control pain. Dr. Cundiff, a cancer pain specialist, says he was invited by the cancer specialty examining board to write for the 1995 exam the first questions about pain management. "There was no category on the exam that dealt with hospice or pain control into which I could fit my questions," claims Cundiff. "We don't need a law to legalize assisted suicide," Dr. Cundiff told me, "we need a law to teach doctors how to treat pain."

Dr. Cundiff could not be more correct when he argues that physicians need better education in controlling the pain experienced by their dying patients. Yet Renee Sahm had excellent control of her pain and still chose suicide to avoid the agonizing hallucinations and confusion that plagued her final weeks of life. And as her throat swelled from the cancer, Renee lived in fear of drowning in her own saliva if the time arrived when she could not swallow at all. "If I continue inhaling through my nostrils, I'm OK," said Renee. "But if I breathe through my mouth I have these horrible spasms of coughing, and the phlegm nearly chokes me to death. I'm so afraid that's the way I'll die."

Mary Hall experienced pain only when she moved about in bed; she did not take her Seconal overdose to escape from poorly treated pain. "It's ridiculous and humiliating for me to stay around anymore," said Mary. "We've all had our say, there's no quality left in my life, and there is nothing left that I need to do. So I'm going."

"Terminally ill people wanting euthanasia or suicide cite pain as the chief factor driving them to want to end their lives," claims Dr. Cundiff. But suffering can entail a lot more than pain: indignity, confusion, disorientation, sedation, immobility, the need for constant care, boredom, loneliness, lying in your own excrement, inability to function on any level that allows enjoyment, simple emotional anguish, fear—all are reasons that have caused people to request euthanasia.

Dr. Cundiff does acknowledge the importance of caring for spiritual as well as physical pain, suggesting that if people can keep busy they will do better with their spiritual suffering. "Writing, reading, and painting," suggests Cundiff, "are all good medicines . . . Sigmund Freud had cancer of the jaw for sixteen years but diverted his attention from his discomfort by writing about psychoanalysis." Both Sigmund Freud and Mary Hall would agree with Dr. Cundiff that writing helped them keep at bay the psychological anguish of their disease. But Freud and Mary Hall had something else in common as well. When Dr. Freud became too sick to write, and when after thirty-three operations the dying bone in his jaw began to smell so bad that even his dog avoided coming near him, Freud stated, "Now it is nothing but torture, and it makes no sense anymore." At Freud's request, his doctor euthanized him with an overdose of morphine.

Since he runs a cancer pain consultation service, it is no wonder that Dr. Cundiff has more experience in treating physical than psychological pain. And there is no doubt that the best in pain management should be the first thing offered to every dying patient who asks for assistance in suicide. But Cundiff claims that adequate pain control can be achieved for virtually all patients as they approach death.

Dr. Timothy Quill, who for eight years ran a hospice in Rochester, New York, and is the author of *Death and Dignity*, has come to different conclusions from those of Dr. Cundiff. "Although I know we have measures to help control pain and lessen suffering," says Dr. Quill, "to think that people do not suffer in the process of dying is an illusion . . . Unfortunately, some patients still experience anguishing deaths in spite of heroic efforts by skilled physicians, nurses, and family members. I am deeply troubled by our profession's unwillingness to openly acknowledge its limitations."

Quill and Cundiff, both physicians with extensive experience in caring for the dying, typify the split that is beginning to tear at the hospice movement. Cundiff claims that if physicians received adequate training, all pain of dying could be adequately controlled. Quill not only disagrees but worries that if doctors do not acknowledge that some of their patients continue to experience unbearable suffering, people will have no alternative but to turn to their families for help to die if they can't stand the agony. Medical ethicist Margaret Pabst Battin, who has done extensive studies on issues around terminal illness, puts it bluntly: "Complete, universal, fully reliable pain control is a myth."

Yet other prominent hospice physicians join with Dr. Cundiff in insisting they can alleviate *all* pain. Dr. Ira Byock, cochair of the Ethics Committee of the Academy of Hospice Physicians, claims that he is "on firm ground in stating that all physical suffering can be controlled . . ." Dr. Byock does acknowledge that for some patients every effort to alleviate pain and suffering fails. But for these unfortunate people, advanced hospice care offers yet another alternative: general anesthesia. When all else fails, proposes Dr. Byock, hospice physicians should use general anesthetics—as if the patient were about to have surgery—to place the dying person in a comatose state until their natural death occurs, days or weeks later.

It is certain that placing dying patients under prolonged and deep anesthesia would relieve their symptoms. But many experts claim that this practice, increasingly being used by hospice physicians today, is virtually the same as killing the patient. Residing in a deep, drug-induced coma while awaiting death can be, from the patient's point of view, no different from death itself.

But Dr. Byock believes that for the family of the patient, this prolonged comatose state can have significant advantages. He recommends that while the patient is under prolonged general anesthesia awaiting a natural death, the family should participate in his or her care. "[I]n the turning and washing . . . family members are called to honor the person departing," states Byock. "I submit that this type of continuing care is a mature, balanced expression for the inner turmoil—the grief—that we may feel."

"I know Ira Byock, and I think he has a goodness and compassion about him," says Dr. Gary Johanson, who sits on the board of the Academy of Hospice Physicians at which Dr. Byock cochairs the ethics committee. "But I don't think Ira's using any sense of logic when he proposes that there is value to be gained in attending to a patient whom we have made comatose to relieve their suffering. The whole thing reflects Ira's value system, and I just don't see how he expects every person on earth to have the same value system that he does. Ira Byock can define for Ira Byock how he wants to die—he can't define it for you or me."

Mary Hall and her family did not need Dr. Byock to advise them of the route to a "mature, balanced expression" for their inner turmoil. They found their own path. "I'm grateful for the last days with you," Mary told her family. "But there is nothing more for us to gain, and I simply will not lay in this bed for the next few days waiting to wither away and die.''

• • •

With all this contentious debate among hospice physicians about euthanasia, it seems strange that they have forgotten that it was hospice philosophy that first broke the ground that made euthanasia acceptable. The difference lies in two words: ''passive'' and ''active.''

When a person is near death and there is no longer hope for cure, hospice agrees with—and encourages—the withdrawal of medical treatments that would prolong life. This ''passive euthanasia'' or ''passive suicide'' is a widely accepted practice today. Cancer patients can spurn further chemotherapy, reject intravenous feedings, decline antibiotics to treat fatal infections, and refuse to be put on breathing machines if a pneumonia overwhelms their lungs—and hospice would not debate the ethics of their acceptance of death. People at the end of a terminal illness who choose to die by refusing further medical intervention are considered to be rational, and their choice is legally and morally acceptable. Within one month in 1994, Richard Nixon, following a stroke, and Jacqueline Onassis, suffering from pneumonia as a complication of cancer, died soon after they refused further medical treatment that could have prolonged their lives but not prevented further suffering. No one questioned their decisions.

Even the Catholic Church, perhaps the world's staunchest opponent of euthanasia, wrote in the 1980 Vatican *Declaration on Euthanasia,* ''When inevitable death is imminent . . . it is permitted in conscience to make the decision to refuse forms of treatment that would only secure a precarious and burdensome prolongation of life.'' Yet when it comes to actively helping someone with a terminal illness to die, Pope John Paul II declared categorically that ''No one can in any way permit the killing of an innocent human being suffering from an incurable disease, or a person who is dying." And the Pope's *Doctrine of the Faith: Declaration on Euthanasia* extended this prohibition to the patients themselves: "Furthermore, no one is permitted to ask for this act of killing."

To hospice, and for the Catholic Church and other religious groups, there is a major moral difference between passively withholding treatment until death ensues and taking action that would help a person to die. To others involved in the care of terminal patients, allowing passive euthanasia by withdrawal of treatment while not also offering active help in dying represents an act of cruelty.

Nancy Cruzan remained in a deep coma after being injured in a car accident when she was twenty-five years old. For seven years, unaware of the world around her, she was kept alive by means of a feeding tube surgically placed in her stomach. When Nancy's parents asked for the feeding tube to be removed to allow their daughter to die, the courts agreed with their "right to refuse medical treatment." One description of the death of Nancy Cruzan after the feeding tube was withdrawn reads as follows: "Family members kept the vigil and watched as she slowly died of dehydration. Nancy's lips dried and blistered. Her tongue grew sticky and swollen, and her eyelids dried and began to stick shut. Toward the end, her breathing grew more labored and raspy with each lung-parching breath of dry hospital air she took." It took eleven days for Nancy Cruzan to die. Had anyone lifted a finger to shorten that process of her inevitable death, to move from passive to active euthanasia by injecting a drug that would have ended Nancy's life, it would have been—and still is by today's laws—murder.

Ethicist Margaret Pabst Battin sees it differently: "If the patient's condition is so tragic . . . then the more merciful act is not one that merely removes support for bodily processes and waits for eventual death to ensue; rather, it is one that brings the pain—and the patient's life—to an end now."

If the final ethical goal is to minimize the suffering of dying, it is clear that active euthanasia is more likely to decrease the final agony than is passively allowing the patient to die. "Letting a disease kill you," says Pabst Battin, "in all the ways that diseases can do that, has the potential to be far more painful, and to involve far more suffering . . . than having a skilled physician bring about your death in a way that is direct, painless, and of the form you want."

While many understandably argue that the decision to actively end someone's life is "playing God," philosopher James Rachels also points out that "If it is for God alone to decide when we shall live and when we shall die, then we 'play God' just as much when we cure people . . .' "

Yet perhaps we don't need to turn to ethicists like Pabst Battin or philosophers like Rachels for the answer to this question. Suicide expert George Howe Colt was told by an elderly woman he interviewed: "When I can't digest my food, when I can't breathe on my own, when my heart can't beat on its own, it could just be that God is trying to tell me something."

Yet for many the distinction between passively waiting for someone to die and actively helping the process along comprises a crucial moral leap between acceptable death and murder. For others, the difference seems no more than an argumentative splitting of hairs; either way, the patient will soon be dead. But the major difference today between passive and active euthanasia is that people who believe in passive euthanasia are allowed to have it; for those who would choose active euthanasia, it is forbidden.

● ● ●

On November 5, 1992, Dr. Timothy Quill, along with Dr. Christine Cassel and Dr. Diane Meier, broke ranks with the policy of the National Hospice Organization and published a paper in the prestigious *New England Journal of Medicine* advocating for the right of physicians to assist in the suicides of their patients. Quill and his colleagues felt they had found a compromise that would satisfy those on both sides of the debate between passive and active euthanasia.

The proposal was simple. Since active participation on the part of a doctor in administering a lethal dose of medication remained ethically uncertain, Quill, Cassel, and Meier proposed that physicians should be allowed to prescribe a lethal amount of a barbiturate such as Seconal to dying patients who asked for it. This would avoid the potential for "error, coercion, or abuse," they claimed, because "ultimately, the patient must be the one to act or not to act." Quill and his colleagues held that the prescribing of a lethal dose of medication was not active euthanasia, since the physician would not physically participate in the patient's death. This midway position, they claimed, would leave the choice between a natural or an accelerated death to each individual person.

The Quill proposal was hotly debated in the medical literature and hailed by many as a compromise position that might be acceptable to both sides of the contentious debate.* But sixteen months later, Mary Hall unwittingly showed why Quill's proposal simply could not work.

"You stay," Mary had told me after her family left the room. "We've got a job to do."

Mary put one of the Seconal tablets in her mouth at a time, then swallowed it with a few gulps of water. Within a few minutes, she had taken nearly all thirty capsules, with a cup-and-a-half of water. When she placed the final pill in her

* In November of 1994, the people of Oregon voted to legalize this very plan in their state, allowing physicians to prescribe lethal dosages of oral medications, but continuing the prohibition against doctors offering other medical help in the suicides of their terminally ill patients.

mouth she looked at me, nodded, and swallowed it down. Then she lay back on the pillow and stared straight ahead, waiting.

For ten minutes, Mary said nothing. Then suddenly, "I'm going to throw up." Mary's voice was calm, but her face showed the panic. She began to repeat, sternly, "I will not vomit, I cannot vomit." But her body was racked with a single convulsive movement as her stomach contracted, propelling its contents upwards. I grabbed a basin and held it in front of her. Mary's hand held my wrist, her grip tight and desperate as she clenched her teeth together to keep the vomit in her mouth from coming out. Then she closed her eyes, tilted her head, and swallowed the pills back down.

A few minutes later, the nausea had passed. "Now there's a trick that's not in *Final Exit*," said Mary. "Tell Derek I wouldn't recommend it." She lay her head back again and slept. Two hours later, she was dead.

"In point of fact," Dr. Quill told me four months after Mary died, "[for a physician to perform] euthanasia for the patient is probably a more humane act than simply giving them the pills to do their own suicide. It's a disaster when people reach a point where they've gone through the whole process, made the decision, taken the pills, and then something happens and it doesn't work."

Quill readily acknowledged that his plan to merely provide patients with pills had its inherent problems. It excludes people who are too weak to take the pills, or forces them to shorten their lives by acting while they still have the strength to do so. And prescribing pills also discriminates against patients with certain types of cancer: Someone with a tumor of the esophagus and no ability to swallow would be denied the same right to assisted suicide granted to a person at the end of her struggle against breast cancer—still able to swallow pills.

And the ethics become fuzzy. Why is death by an oral

medication more ethically clean and acceptable than death by an injected medication? "Perhaps the most fundamental commitment that physicians make to their dying patients," wrote Dr. Quill in his book *Death and Dignity,* "is not to abandon them, no matter how the last stages of their illness may unfold . . . The profession appears to turn its back in these horrible moments in order to keep its intentions pure."

And yet Quill and his colleagues' proposal to prescribe lethal medications but never to physically aid in their administration does make doctors turn their backs on those patients who choose an assisted death but are too weak or unable to swallow. And if a patient should vomit the pills, the doctor could do no more than stand by and say, "I'm sorry, but it seems you're one of those for whom this method will not work."

The Quill plan, as bold as it was in publicly opposing the firm opposition of the National Hospice Organization, had another major flaw, perhaps more important than all other drawbacks. It provided inadequate safeguards to assure that the patients who were taking the overdose of prescribed pills had first been offered the utmost in the care of their pain and suffering before they decided to kill themselves.

Assisted suicide, active euthanasia, and even passive euthanasia should be available only to patients who have first had the fullest chance to control the suffering of dying by every possible means other than by bringing on their own death. And there is only one group of physicians and nurses qualified, experienced, and knowledgeable enough to be certain that dying patients have been offered the best care before they choose to take their lives: those who have been trained in and practice the methods of hospice.

• • •

Two weeks before Pierre died, Gordon sat in the living room of his apartment, watching the movie *JFK.* Pierre had become extremely weak, sleeping almost the entire day, and Gordon was sure he was soundly asleep in the bedroom. At the end of the long film, Gordon got up from the couch and saw that the light on the answering machine of his separate phone line was blinking: one message. He flipped on the recording. "Gordon, where are you?" Pierre's voice was barely audible on the machine. Gordon rushed to his side. "Pierre actually didn't need anything," he recalled. "He was just lonely and wanted me to check on him."

"Sometimes all that hospice can offer," said Clarissa, "is to be there. People know we have a lot of experience with the dying, and it just makes them less frightened of the whole thing if we're around."

For Pierre, hospice offered much more than a persistent presence. "After my first meeting with Pierre," recalled Clarissa, "I walked out of there thinking, 'Oh, God, do I ever have to go back there again? This is so depressing!' He was one of the most hopeless cases I had ever confronted in terms of attitude and depression. And there was no doubt that he had plans for suicide. I knew all of this; and I also knew there was so much that hospice had to offer him—the least of which was that we made it possible for him to be cared for at home instead of at the hospital."

"If Pierre had stayed at the hospital," added Gordon, "he would have killed himself no matter what I said, or Stephen, or Lynn, or even Alexa."

"Actually," thought Clarissa, "he wouldn't have been kept at the hospital, it would have been a nursing home. Imagine Pierre in a nursing home?"

While the initial benefit of hospice for Pierre was simply to get him back home from the hospital, when his illness progressed Clarissa's work became far more specific.

"In the last few weeks," she recalled, "Pierre had infections and fluid in his lungs. He became very short of breath, and he was tremendously frightened that he would die while fighting to breathe. And, God, that is scary! But we were able to reassure him, get him oxygen to use at home, teach him how to work with his breathing, give him low doses of morphine to relax his diaphragm and relieve his sensation of suffocation. We even put a fan in his room to be sure he'd feel air circulating around him. There was so much to offer him. And we got him past his fear.''

Time after time, Clarissa and the hospice aides worked out thoughtful and complex ways to make Pierre's dying days more comfortable and less frightening. While Alexa may have been responsible for helping Pierre over the first hump of his depression, there is no doubt that the skilled and caring attention from the hospice workers kept him from killing himself after Alexa was gone and his illness progressed.

"Pierre went through this revolution,'' said Clarissa, "and we happened to be fortunate enough to be a part of it. It's our goal to have patients be at peace with what is happening, and Pierre really achieved that. And just because I've seen lots of deaths that weren't as good as Pierre's doesn't mean I don't believe in hospice. Hospice care is still the best that can be offered to a patient who is dying. I just wish everyone had the chance at it.''

Clarissa Ramstead has no special training in medical ethics, philosophy, or how to write laws. But a leap can be made from her compassionate desire to offer the best of care to everyone who is dying, to a law that would incorporate the best of the philosophies of hospice and Hemlock. A system could be developed so that when any patient who is near death asks for assistance in suicide or for active euthanasia, a hospice physician and nurse are rapidly made available to evaluate the patient's care and to offer the patient and family the best of their skills. If patients are requesting aid in suicide because, like Pierre in his final weeks, they fear a death while fighting to breathe, hospice can assure them that there are methods to help. And if the patient is asking for death because of poorly controlled pain, the hospice team could have their best try at decreasing that patient's pain.

But integral to this plan would be an understanding that, if as sometimes will happen, the best efforts of hospice to alleviate a patient's suffering fail, and firm and repeated requests to have help to die more quickly continue—then it is the patient's wish, not hospice philosophy, that is finally respected.

There are many good reasons why laws that might legalize physician assistance in suicide have repeatedly been rejected by the public. People want better care in dying before they will grant physicians the right to euthanize them. But today the public is not receiving better care in dying, nor the right to assisted suicide or euthanasia. If a hospice specialist's advice and care became the mandated response to a suffering patient's request for death, no one would be put to death without first being offered the best of care. And no one would be refused death and forced to suffer on should they persistently say, "Enough."

• • •

On July 14, 1994, only twenty months after Dr. Quill proposed that physicians should be permitted to write lethal prescriptions for dying patients, and just four months after the death of Mary Hall, Quill joined with five other physicians in a new article in the *New England Journal of Medicine* and reversed his entire position—deciding that merely prescribing pills was not sufficient, and that doctors should be able to participate in active euthanasia.

"I knew that limitations existed in the first plan," said Dr. Quill when I called him, surprised to hear about his turn-around. "I knew we'd been making some arbitrary distinction between who could be helped and who couldn't—and that that wouldn't hold up for long. But we hadn't come up with the safeguards at that time to go any further with it. Now, we've designed the safeguards, and I believe that active euthanasia is simply the kinder process if we're going to help certain patients to die."

The safeguards proposed by Dr. Quill and his colleagues in their new proposal involve using "palliative care" specialists to evaluate the treatment of any patient who is requesting euthanasia. "Palliative care" simply refers to the process of treating terminal patients to relieve their symptoms rather than cure their diseases. The method has also come to be called "comfort care." In this country, virtually all palliative care specialists have received their training in hospices, worked in hospices, or are still hospice physicians. In fact, Dr. Quill defines "comfort care" as "palliative and supportive treatment used in hospice programs and elsewhere."

The new Quill plan proposes to use palliative care experts to review *all* requests for assisted suicide or euthanasia. The specialist in comfort care would talk with the patient and primary physician, and review the medical records and treatments that have already been used. And if the palliative care specialist agrees that all possibilities for hospice-style comfort and symptom relief have been tried and have failed (or at least been offered and rejected by the patient), the palliative care physician, backed by a review committee, could then authorize physician-assisted suicide or active euthanasia for that patient.

But if the palliative care doctor finds that the patient's request for euthanasia comes from inadequate treatment of his symptoms, wrote Quill and his colleagues, "The process of consultation might lead to improved pain management or the use of other means of comfort care." In any case, a patient who had not yet received adequate comfort care would be offered better treatment of symptoms, not death.

"If this plan is accepted," Quill told me, "we'll be able to accommodate whichever method is most consistent with each patient's values, to provide for the most humane death. Everyone who wants euthanasia will be offered the best of comfort care first. And for those for whom it simply cannot work, and who want to die sooner rather than continue to suffer, we'll be able to help them as well."

Quill's new proposal makes sense, but it may be offering too little too late by requiring the aid of a comfort care specialist only when a dying patient has reached such a point of desperation that he requests assistance in suicide.

It would be better to go one step further: *All* dying patients should be offered the option of palliative care expertise, that is, hospice care—*before* they are driven by their misery to ask for help in suicide. If hospice practitioners are as good as they say they are, and there is every indication that this is true, then fewer patients would ever reach the point of asking to be put to death.

The cost of hospice care in the home of a terminally ill patient averages about eighty dollars per day. And good hospice care avoids repeated hospitalizations—which cost thousands of dollars—for patients in distress at the end of life. There is sound moral, medical, and economic sense to making hospice care a uniform benefit provided by insurance companies, hospitals, or whatever new "universal coverage" plan the government finally provides for its citizens. And if the principles of Dame Cecily Saunders can be offered to every dying patient, most requests for euthanasia will, as her advocates claim, disappear.

But for some, and no one can predict how many there will be, even the best of hospice care will not work. For those, a palliative care specialist trained to evaluate requests for euthanasia would be called in. And the patient would again receive the chance of better treatment of her suffering before being offered death. In the end, though, for all patients, the choice would be theirs.

Such a system of "hospice and Hemlock" would offer all dying patients the reassurance that their individual choices would be respected, and that the best skills in helping them to die comfortably—by whichever method—would be available.

"Let's put it this way," observed Clarissa. "I think if assisted suicide and euthanasia are going to become legal someday, hospice needs to be involved. Before someone is given the choice of suicide, they should also be given the chance for a good natural death. And hospice workers have more knowledge in managing pain, suffering, and fears, and in focusing on spiritual as well as physical needs, than anyone else. So first let me try everything that all of my experience as a hospice nurse has taught me, and I'll make most people feel better without having to kill themselves. Let me do that first—but then we should respect whatever decision they make about how they want to die and help them in any way we can."

• • •

With public pressure and with the appropriate safeguards in place, hospice and Hemlock could someday combine their philosophies and practices, based on their shared ambition to help people achieve the best death possible. But today, patients who are concerned about the way they may die face a medical system filled with secrecy, contradictions, contentious debate, and at times outright hypocrisy. If the public is concerned about the unfairness and abuses that may occur if assisted suicide and euthanasia were made legal, they might well look at the system as it is working now.

Derek Humphry recently received a note from his publisher proudly proclaiming that the sales figures for *Final Exit* had grown from 520,000 to 645,000. Every month well over one thousand people still buy his book of recipes for suicide. And Humphry's pamphlet about the best way to use a plastic bag in "self-deliverance" continues to be his organization's bestselling informational leaflet.

In Michigan, Dr. Jack Kevorkian, a pathologist with no experience in medical care of people with terminal illnesses, has carried on a campaign to change the laws prohibiting assisted suicide by putting to death twenty people he barely knew.

In an informal survey at the University of Chicago Hospital, Dr. Christine Cassel repeatedly asked her fellow physicians about how they would like to die. Even doctors who firmly opposed the legalization of assisted suicide and euthanasia told Cassel that "when my time comes" they would use their ability to obtain deadly drugs to end their lives if they were suffering. Their patients, of course, do not share this option.

And in the past two years, I had come to know Renee Sahm, Pierre Nadeau, Gene Robbins, Kelly Niles, and Mary Hall—and watched in horror as they and their families confronted the issue of assisted suicide as it occurs under today's legal prohibition.

Clarissa Ramstead, intent on dealing with Pierre's spiritual as well as his physical illness, could not talk with him about his specific plans for suicide. "I just won't keep it hidden like that anymore," Clarissa told me recently. "Basically, I've decided to break the rules. I tell my patients, 'Let's talk about it.' "

When Mary Hall made her final decision to die by an overdose of Seconal, her son-in-law had to guard the door in case the nurses might come in and stop her. And Mary endured the final indignity of swallowing her own vomit in order to achieve her desire for a prompt death.

Gene Robbins found his expert in death and dying by calling the Hemlock Society and meeting Sarah. Four weeks later he lay at home with a plastic bag around his head.

In agony, Joan Agnes McMahon read through *Final Exit* and planned a way to end the life of her son, Kelly, who finally defied the prohibition against assisted suicide by starving himself to death.

And on March 28, 1993, I sat alone beside an unconscious Renee Sahm and confronted the question of whether or not to help my friend achieve the death she had chosen.

•   •   •

My father, now seventy-six, has had two heart attacks. My mother at seventy-five continues to suffer from depression and inflammatory bowel disease. She has also had a series of small strokes. It will not be long, I know, before they approach their deaths. When they do, the first action I will take is to contact a hospice team for help and guidance in their care. And that will probably be enough.

But if hospice cannot ease the torture of their dying, I know my parents will call on me to help. "Lonny, I had no one else to turn to," said my mother when I was fourteen. I pray that if my own father or mother repeatedly cries out for relief, it will not fall on me to respond to their pleas and administer the pills, inject the medication, or use a plastic bag to end their suffering. I want at my side a hospice physician and nurse who will offer them the best of care. And if that is not enough, these health professionals should be able openly to arrange an injection that would provide my parents with the most merciful death.

When I sat with Mary's son Paul and his wife and child in the backyard of their Southern California home, I felt a chill as he said to me, "If the doctors wouldn't do it, I would have helped Mom die. But it would be the most painful thing for the rest of my life—what a horrible thing for a son to have to do." Then Paul continued. "Can't we find a better way to help people who are dying?"

A F T E R W O R D

A*Chosen Death* was published in August 1995, its final paragraphs filled with my concerns about how we die, ending with a meditation on the eventual deaths of my own parents.

On June 19, 1996, my mother died without warning of a heart attack, ending our dance around assisted suicide that had begun when I was fourteen and she'd asked me to inject her with a lethal dose of potassium chloride. I mourned her, and breathed a sigh of relief that we had ended the dance without tragedy.

But death had other plans. On July 8, 1997, three hours after the United States Supreme Court proclaimed that dying patients had no right to assistance should they wish to hasten their deaths, my father died.

That is, his brain died. His body did not die until the next day, and then only because he and I had long ago come to a different conclusion than that reached by the nine justices of the Supreme Court about his right to die in the way he chose.

By the time I raced across the country to his side in the Intensive Care Unit, he was in a deep coma, kept alive with a machine that breathed for him, and IVs to keep his blood circulating. Neither, however, made his brain function.

But we had done all the right things: signed the Living Will and the Durable Power of Attorney; discussed as a family the toughest questions about how we might die, and under what circumstances we would not want to live. "If . . . there can be no recovery from such condition that my death is imminent," reads my father's living will, "I direct that life-prolonging procedures be withheld or withdrawn."

Within a few hours of my arrival, the physicians, nurses, myself and, I am certain, my father, all agreed that the machinery should be disconnected, the tubes removed. The articulated intent, by every one of us, was for my father to die.

When the machinery had been turned off, *intent* soon became the key word—for my dad showed no signs that he was about to die, not at that moment, possibly not for days, possibly not until starvation and dehydration would finally beat his heart into submission. For hours, he lay sweating, gasping for breath, gurgling—but not dying.

We had intended for him to die.

"Please," I turned to the nurse, "ask the doctor for an order to heavily sedate him, to stop the agony of this prolonged suffocation."

"We can't do that," she replied, and the debate, much shorter than the arguments I'd heard at the Supreme Court, was over.

Although we had intended for my father to die when we turned off the life support machines, his continued breathing had changed the rules: We could not legally administer medications intending to cause his death.

I kept the vigil for hours, caressed his soaking forehead, whispered loving words to ease his torturous breathing and let his suffering end. The volume of my tears equaled that of the sweat drenching his hospital gown. But the rattling of his breathing drowned out my crying. And then I could abandon him no longer.

"Excuse me," I said to the nurse, "my father and I need to be alone."

With the doors closed, we had one more father-son conversation about the Supreme Court decision. "It seems that you and I and the justices," I said, my cheek against his, holding him in my arms, "have a difference of opinion as to how you should die. I know whose opinion to follow at this moment."

Five minutes later, when the alarms from his heart monitor shrilled, announcing that his breathing and heartbeat had stopped, no one responded. My dad lay in my arms, the two of us alone, in peace.

My dear, good justices, you have listened to the best arguments of both sides. And I know you have completed your work, your decision behind you.

But I ask you now to listen to one more voice, that of Irving Shavelson, my father, who died on June 27, some twenty hours after you proclaimed that states can forbid hastening a terminally ill patient's death.

Alone, I faced the irony, the tears, and the anguish of how he died. Will you now join me in listening to Irving Shavelson, should you again consider whether it is a dying person and his family, or fifty different state legislatures, who should be in our rooms dictating the rules as our last breaths are gasped?

ACKNOWLEDGMENTS

With my most heartfelt appreciation to Renee Sahm, Pierre Nadeau, Gene Robbins, Kelly Niles, and Mary Hall. I miss you all. And to the families and friends of each, who became my friends as well.

• • •

Warmest thanks to Fred Setterberg, who somehow manages to juggle being mentor, colleague and close friend, all at the same time. My gratitude to the many others who stuck it out through a rough two years of my repeatedly becoming close to people who were soon to die: Kim Bancroft, Deborah Bickel, Renee Emunah, Susan Foster, Loralie Froman, Susan and David Glanville, Charles Hale, Carol Jenkins, April Rapier, Amy Shapiro, Melissa Smith, Ann Van Steenberg, and the Emergency Department staff at Alta Bates Hospital. And to Darrel Hunt, Steve Shiflett, and John Chidester—who taught me about how the gay community is dealing with the issue of assisted suicide, and who have all since died of AIDS.

• • •

Special gratitude to those who worked on both the words and photographs in this book: Wendy Ledger and Paul Marcus.

• • •

And thanks for the support and encouragement from *Impact Visuals,* David Friend at *Life,* David France at *Lear's,* Dave Rummel and Reid Orvedahl at ABC News' *Turning Point.*

• • •

Finally, sincere gratitude for their hard work and talent to my literary agent, Felicia Eth, and my editor at Simon & Schuster, Bob Bender.

BIBLIOGRAPHY

Alvarez, A. *The Savage God. A Study of Suicide.* New York: Random House, 1972.

Angell, M. "Don't Criticize Dr. Death." *New York Times,* 14 June 1990, A14.

Annas, George J., J.D., M.P.H. "Physician-Assisted Suicide—Michigan's Temporary Solution." *Legal Issues in Medicine* 328, no. 21 (27 May 1993): 1573.

Batavia, Andrew I. "A Disability Rights–Independent Living Perspective on Euthanasia." *Western Journal of Medicine* 154, no. 5 (May 1991): 153.

Benrubi, Guy I., M.D. "Sounding Board: Euthanasia—The Need for Procedural Safeguards." *New England Journal of Medicine* (16 January 1992): Letters.

Blendon, Robert J., et al. "Should Physicians Aid Their Patients in Dying?" *Journal of the American Medical Association* 267 (20 May 1992): 2658.

Brody, Howard, M.D., Ph.D. "Assisted Death: A Compassionate Response to a Medical Failure." *New England Journal of Medicine* (5 November 1992): 1384.

Brody, Jane. "Doctors Admit Ignoring Dying Patient's Wishes." *New York Times*, 14 January 1993, A12.

Burnell, George M., M.D. *Final Choices: To Live or to Die, in an Age of Medical Technology*. New York: Plenum Press, 1993.

Byock, Ira R., M.D. "Consciously Walking the Fine Line: Thoughts on a Hospice Response to Assisted Suicide and Euthanasia." *Journal of Palliative Care* 9, no. 3 (1993): 25–28.

———. "The Euthanasia/Assisted Suicide Debate Matures." *The American Journal of Hospice and Palliative Care* (March/April 1993): 8.

———. "Final Exit: A Wake-Up Call to Hospice." *The Hospice Journal* 7, no. 4 (1991): 51.

Camus, Albert. *The Myth of Sisyphus and Other Essays*. New York: Knopf, 1955.

Cassel, Christine. "The Popular Movement for Physician-Assisted Dying—What the Public Is Saying, What Physicians Are Hearing." *Western Journal of Medicine* 157 (August 1992): 191.

Cassel, Christine K., M.D., and Diane E. Meier, M.D. "Sounding Board: Morals and Moralism in the Debate Over Euthanasia and Assisted Suicide." *New England Journal of Medicine* (13 September 1990): 750.

Charmaz, Cathy. *The Social Reality of Death*. New York: Addison-Wesley, 1980.

Colt, George Howe. *The Enigma of Suicide: A Timely Investigation into the Causes, the Possibilities for Prevention and the Paths to Healing*. New York: Simon & Schuster, 1991.

Cundiff, David, M.D. *Euthanasia Is Not the Answer: A Hospice Physician's View*. Totawa, N.J.: Humana Press, 1992.

Davis, Thomas N., III, M.D. *No Final Exit: A Psychiatrist's Rebuttal—Guidance for True Deliverance and Renewed Life*. Fletcher, N.C.: New Puritan Library, 1992.

Dawson, John. "Last Rites and Wrongs—Euthanasia: Autonomy and Responsibility." *Cambridge Quarterly of Healthcare Ethics* 1 (1992): 81–83.

Dougherty, Margot, and Sandra Rubin Tessler. "Tiring of Life Without Freedom, Quadriplegic David Rivlin Chooses to Die Among Friends." *USA Today*, 21 July 1989; also 7 July 1989.

Dworkin, Ronald. "When Is It Right to Die?" *New York Times*, 17 May 1994, A19.

Dyck, Arthur J. "An Alternative to the Ethic of Euthanasia." In *Ethics in Medicine: Historical Perspectives and Contemporary Concerns*, edited by Stanley Joel Reiser, Arthur J. Dyck and William J. Curran. Cambridge: MIT Press, 1977.

Fadiman, Anne. "Death News: Requiem for the *Hemlock Quarterly*." *Harper's*, April 1994, 74–78.

Foley, Kathleen M., M.D. "The Relationship of Pain and Symptom Management to Patient Requests for Physician Assisted Suicide." *Journal of Pain and Symptom Management* 6, no. 5 (July 1991): 289.

Fye, W. Bruce. "Active Euthanasia: An Historical Survey of Its Conceptual Origins and Introduction Into Medical Thought." *Bulletin. The History of Medicine* (1979): 492–502.

Gabriel, Trip. "A Fight to the Death: Was Ann Humphry's 'Final Exit' intended to pull the plug on her ex-husband's right-to-die movement?" *New York Times Magazine*, 8 December 1991.

Girsh, Faye J., Ed.D. "Physician Aid in Dying—What Physicians Say, What Patients Say." *Western Journal of Medicine* 157 (August 1992): 188–9.

Gross, Jane. "At AIDS Epicenter, Seeking Swift, Sure Death." *New York Times*, 20 June 1993.

Hoefler, James M., and Brian E. Kamoie. *Deathright: Culture, Medicine, Politics, and the Right to Die*. Boulder, Colo.: Westview Press, 1994.

Humphry, Derek. *Dying With Dignity: What You Need to Know About Euthanasia*. New York: St. Martin's, 1992.

————. *Final Exit: The Practicalities of Self-Deliverance and Assisted Suicide for the Dying*. New York: Dell, 1991.

————. *Lawful Exit: The Limits of Freedom for Help in Dying*. Junction City, Ore.: Norris Lane Press, 1993.

————. *Let Me Die Before I Wake*. Revision of 1982 book. Eugene, Ore.: Hemlock Society, 1986.

―――. "Open Forum." *San Francisco Chronicle*, 13 November 1992.

―――. Advertisement about the death of Ann Humphry. *New York Times*, 14 October 1991.

Johnson, Mary. "Drab Curtains: Or How the Press Didn't Cover the Issues That Led to David Rivlin's Suicide." *The Disability Rag*, September 1989, 23.

Kevorkian, Jack. *Prescription Medicide: The Goodness of a Planned Death.* Buffalo, N.Y.: Prometheus Books, 1991.

Kolata, Gina. "Saying Life Is Not Enough: The Disabled Demand Rights and Choices." *New York Times*, 31 January 1991.

Longmore, Paul K. "Assisted Suicide—What Euthanasia Activists Say, What People With Disabilities Say." *Western Journal of Medicine* 157, no. 2 (August 1992): 190.

―――. "To Live, to Die—Who Decides?: The Strange Death of David Rivlin." *Western Journal of Medicine* 157, no. 2 (May 1991): 154.

Mair, George B. *How to Die With Dignity.* Scottish EXIT, 1980.

Marzuk, Peter M., et al. "Increase in Suicide by Asphyxiation in New York City After the Publication of *Final Exit.*" *New England Journal of Medicine* (11 November 1993): 1508.

Miller, John, ed. *On Suicide: Great Writers on the Ultimate Question.* San Francisco: Chronicle Books, 1992.

Miller, Robert J. "Hospice Care: An Alternative to Euthanasia." *Law, Medicine, and Health Care* 20:I-2 (Spring/Summer 1992): 128.

Miller, Franklin, et al. "Sounding Board: Regulating Physician-Assisted Death." *New England Journal of Medicine* (14 July 1994): 119.

Nuland, Sherwin B. *How We Die: Reflections on Life's Final Chapter.* New York: Knopf, 1994.

Olszewski, Lori. "Hospice Movement Offers Alternative to Hospital Death." *San Francisco Chronicle*, 20 October 1992.

Orentlicher, D. "Physician Participation in Assisted Suicide." *Journal of the American Medical Association* 262 (6 October 1989): 1844–5.

Pabst Battin, Margaret. *The Least Worst Death: Essays on Bioethics on the End of Life.* New York: Oxford University Press, 1994.

Pace, Nicholas, M.D. Letter to editor: "We Should Treat Depression, Not Assist Suicide." *New York Times,* 4 February 1993.

Quill, Timothy, M.D. "The Care of Last Resort." *New York Times,* 23 July 1994.

———. *Death and Dignity: Making Choices and Taking Charge.* New York: Norton, 1993.

———. Editorial. *New York Times,* 27 September 1993.

———. "On Trial: How We Die." *New York Times,* 27 September 1993, Op-Ed.

———. "Sounding Board: Death and Dignity—A Case of Individualized Decision Making." *New England Journal of Medicine* (7 March 1991): 692.

Quill, Timothy E., M.D., Christine Cassel, M.D., and Diane E. Meier, M.D. "Care of the Hopelessly Ill: Proposed Clinical Criteria for Physician Assisted Suicide." *New England Journal of Medicine* (5 November 1992): 1380–5.

Rachels, James. "Active and Passive Euthanasia." *New England Journal of Medicine* (9 January 1975): 78.

Ram Dass and Mirabai Bush. *Compassion in Action: Setting Out on the Path of Service.* New York: Bell Tower, 1992.

Reiser, Stanley Joel. "The Dilemma of Euthanasia in Modern Medical History: The English and American Experience." In *Ethics in Medicine: Historical Perspectives and Contemporary Concerns,* edited by Stanley Joel Reiser, Arthur J. Dyck and William J. Curran. Cambridge: MIT Press, 1977.

Rosenblatt, Stanley M. *Murder of Mercy: Euthanasia on Trial.* Buffalo, N.Y.: Prometheus Books, 1992.

Rosenthal, Elisabeth. "Study Finds Suicides Follow a Book." *New York Times,* 6 November 1993.

Saunders, Dame Cecily. "Caring to the End." *Nursing Mirror,* 4 September 1980.

Singer, Peter A., and Mark Siegler. "Sounding Board: Euthanasia—a Critique." *New England Journal of Medicine* (28 June 1990): 1881.

Solomon, Mildred, M.D. "Decisions Near the End of Life—Professionals' Views on Life-sustaining Treatments." *American Journal of Public Health* 83 (January 1993): 14–23.

Stoddard, Sandol. *The Hospice Movement: A Better Way of Caring for the Dying.* Updated and Expanded. New York: Vintage, 1992.

Twycross, Robert G. "Assisted Death: A Reply." *The Lancet* (29 September 1990): 796.

Wanzer, Sidney H., M.D., et al. "The Physician's Responsibility Toward Hopelessly Ill Patients: A Second Look." *New England Journal of Medicine* (30 March 1989): 844.

Winslade, William J., and Judith Wilson Ross. *Choosing Life or Death.* New York: Free Press, 1986.

Other Articles of Interest

"The Seventeenth Annual Law Review Symposium, 'The Right to Die.' " *Ohio Northern University Law Review* 20, no. 3 (1993).

"Statement of the National Hospice Organization Opposing the Legalization of Euthanasia and Assisted Suicide." Arlington, Va.: National Hospice Organization, 8 November 1990.

Blacks and euthanasia: "Michigan Panel Narrowly Backs Suicide Aid." *New York Times*, 6 March 1994.

Disability and euthanasia: "Unanswered Questions." *The Disability Rag*, September 1990.